Integrative Medicine

Editor

KEVIN K. HAUSSLER

VETERINARY CLINICS OF NORTH AMERICA: EQUINE PRACTICE

www.vetequine.theclinics.com

Consulting Editor
RAMIRO E. TORIBIO

December 2022 • Volume 38 • Number 3

ELSEVIER

1600 John F. Kennedy Boulevard • Suite 1800 • Philadelphia, Pennsylvania, 19103-2899

http://www.vetequine.theclinics.com

VETERINARY CLINICS OF NORTH AMERICA: EQUINE PRACTICE Volume 38, Number 3
December 2022 ISSN 0749-0739, ISBN-13: 978-0-323-84940-1

Editor: Taylor Hayes
Developmental Editor: Ann Gielou Posedio

Veterinary Clinics of North America: Equine Practice (ISSN 0749-0739) is published in April, August, and December by Elsevier Inc., 360 Park Avenue South, New York, NY 10010-1710. Business and Editorial Offices: 1600 John F. Kennedy Blvd., Suite 1800, Philadelphia, PA 19103-2899. Subscription prices are $299.00 per year (domestic individuals), $777.00 per year (domestic institutions), $100.00 per year (domestic students/residents), $341.00 per year (Canadian individuals), $789.00 per year (Canadian institutions), $372.00 per year (international individuals), $789.00 per year (international institutions), $100.00 per year (Canadian students/residents), and $180.00 per year (international students/residents). To receive student/resident rate, orders must be accompanied by name of affiliated institution, date of term, and the signature of program/residency coordinator on institution letterhead. Orders will be billed at individual rate until proof of status is received. Foreign air speed delivery is included in all *Clinics* subscription prices. All prices are subject to change without notice. **POSTMASTER:** Send address changes to *Veterinary Clinics of North America: Equine Practice*, 3251 Riverport Lane, Maryland Heights, MO 63043. Customer Service (orders, claims, online, change of address): Elsevier Health Sciences Division, Subscription **Customer Service, 3251 Riverport Lane, Maryland Heights, MO 63043. Tel: 1-800-654-2452 (U.S. and Canada); 314-447-8871 (outside U.S. and Canada). Fax: 314-447-8029. E-mail: journalscustomerservice-usa@elsevier.com (for print support);** E-mail: **journalsonlinesupport-usa@ elsevier.com (for online support).**

Reprints. For copies of 100 or more of articles in this publication, please contact the Commercial Reprints Department, Elsevier Inc., 360 Park Avenue South, New York, NY 10010-1710. Tel.: 212-633-3874; Fax: 212-633-3820; E-mail: reprints@elsevier.com.

Veterinary Clinics of North America: Equine Practice is covered in *MEDLINE/PubMed (Index Medicus), Excerpta Medica, Current Contents/Agriculture, Biology and Environmental Sciences,* and *ISI*.

Contributors

CONSULTING EDITOR

RAMIRO E. TORIBIO, DVM, MS, PhD
Diplomate, American College of Veterinary Internal Medicine; Professor and Trueman
Endowed Chair of Equine Medicine and Surgery, College of Veterinary Medicine, The Ohio
State University, Columbus, Ohio, USA

EDITOR

KEVIN K. HAUSSLER, DVM, DC, PhD
Diplomate, American College of Veterinary Sports Medicine and Rehabilitation, Associate
Professor, Department of Clinical Sciences, Colorado State University, Fort Collins,
Colorado, USA

AUTHORS

STEVE ADAIR, MS, DVM
Diplomate, American College of Veterinary Surgeons, Diplomate, American College of
Veterinary Sports Medicine and Rehabilitation, Professor of Equine Surgery, Department
of Large Animal Clinical Science, University of Tennessee, College of Veterinary Medicine,
Knoxville, Tennessee, USA

EDWARD BOLDT Jr, DVM
Performance Horse Complementary Medicine Services, PLLC, Fort Collins, Colorado,
USA

HILARY M. CLAYTON, BVMS, PhD
Professor and McPhail Dressage Chair Emerita, Department of Large Animal Clinical
Sciences, College of Veterinary Medicine, Michigan State University, East Lansing,
Michigan, USA; CEO, Sport Horse Science, Mason, Michigan, USA

**LESLEY GOFF, PhD, MANIMST(ANIMPHYSIO), MAPPSC(EXSPSC),
GDIPAPPSC(MANIPPHYSIO), BAPPSC(PHYSIO)**
Adjunct Research Fellow, School of Veterinary Science, University of Queensland,
Director, Active Animal Physiotherapy and Hip Sport Spine Physiotherapy, Highfields,
Queensland, Australia

KEVIN K. HAUSSLER, DVM, DC, PhD
Diplomate, American College of Veterinary Sports Medicine and Rehabilitation, Associate
Professor, Department of Clinical Sciences, Colorado State University, Fort Collins,
Colorado, USA

**KIMBERLY HENNEMAN, DVM, Diplomate ACVSMR (Equine, Canine), CVA (IVAS),
CVC (AVCA)**
Animal Health VIPS (Veterinary Integrative & Performance Specialists), Park City, Utah,
USA

TIM N. HOLT, DVM
Professor, Department of Clinical Sciences, Colorado State University, Fort Collins, Colorado, USA

MELISSA R. KING, DVM, PhD
Diplomate of the American College of Veterinary Sports Medicine and Rehabilitation, Associate Professor, Equine Sports Medicine and Rehabilitation, Colorado State University Veterinary Teaching Hospital, Equine Orthopaedic Research Center, Fort Collins, Fort Collins, Colorado, USA

TUULIA LUOMALA, PT
MT-Physio Oy, Lempäälä, Finland

RUSSELL MACKECHNIE-GUIRE, PhD
Reader, Hartpury University, Gloucestershire, United Kingdom; Director, Centaur Biomechanics, LTD, Dunstaffnage House, Moreton Morrell, Warwickshire, Russell, United Kingdom

EMILY MANGAN, DVM, CTCVMP, CCRV, CVMMP
Wisewood Integrative Veterinary Medicine, LLC, Pleasant Hill, Oregon, USA

JENNIFER REPAC, DVM
Diplomate, American College of Veterinary Sports Medicine and Rehabilitation, Assistant Clinical Professor, University of Florida, College of Veterinary Medicine, Gainesville, Florida, USA

MELINDA R. STORY, DVM, PhD
Diplomate, American College of Veterinary Surgeons, Diplomate, American College of Veterinary Sports Medicine and Rehabilitation, Assistant Professor, Equine Sports Medicine and Rehabilitation, Orthopedic Research Center, C. Wayne McIlwraith Translational Medicine Institute, Department of Clinical Sciences, Colorado State University, Fort Collins, Colorado, USA

HUISHENG XIE, DVM, MS, PhD
Chi University, Reddick, Florida, USA

Contents

Integrative medicine is based on a model of being proactive and promoting health and wellness, rather than being reactive and solely focusing on episodic disease processes. Integrative medicine incorporates a holistic approach to clinical practice that encourages owner involvement with a focus on individualized care, maintained wellness, optimized performance, and disease prevention. Health promotion and preventative care require a different set of clinical skills and perspectives than is typically provided by a traditional veterinary education. Productive interprofessional collaborations are an essential component to the effective delivery of integrative medicine services.

This article serves as an introduction into integrative case management as it applies to the horse's mental health, pain management, and tissue healing. The integrative philosophy pertains to the combination of conventional Western medicine and complementary and alternative therapies to provide the best patient care possible using currently available evidence. The goal is to improve the health of the patient in a more holistic manner.

Addressing poor performance issues in horses is a common yet challenging request to veterinarians. Often, there are limited field diagnostic or therapy choices. Growing lay popularity in integrative therapies, as well as increasing clinical incorporation, is creating more awareness of their clinical applications. Many modalities are showing increasing evidence of positive outcomes with minimal harm, but additional safety and efficacy evaluation is needed. Integrative modalities have unique ways of perceiving disease patterns that are different from more modern approaches, and these different perspectives can be used diagnostically and therapeutically either combined with more conventional approaches, or when those approaches fall short.

Horses 15 years of age and older now account for a significant portion of the equine population. Integrative therapies can provide important diagnostic and treatment tools for managing and maintaining the health of geriatric horses. Aged horses are often afflicted with chronic disease processes that are difficult to effectively manage with conventional medicinal approaches, such as laminitis and osteoarthritis. Diagnostic and therapeutic approaches using integrative therapies, such as acupuncture and spinal manipulation, are presented in this article for managing aged horses with metabolic disorders and musculoskeletal pain, stiffness, or muscle hypertonicity.

Equine cervical pain and dysfunction may be difficult to diagnose and effectively manage. Understanding techniques in integrative medicine often allows the practitioner to observe and palpate areas of pain and dysfunction in the horse being evaluated in ways often not taught or used in conventional medicine. There are many integrative therapies that also may be utilized to more effectively manage these horses, resulting in a more comfortable and functional horse.

 Video content accompanies this article at http://www.vetequine. theclinics.com.

Fascia is a complex and intriguing tissue, which can take on structural properties of being loose or dense, irregular or regular. Fascia functions by connecting, separating, and uniting different structures of the body. Myofascial dysfunction can be a significant source of pain and can be categorized as densification, adhesion, and fibrosis. Digital palpation and treatment of myofascial disorders can be provided via superficial or deep techniques. Different myofascial treatment techniques include slow and fast techniques, which can be applied at different depths, angles, and rhythms.

 Video content accompanies this article at http://www.vetequine. theclinics.com.

There is a growing body of evidence to support the use of spinal mobilization and manipulation techniques in equine practice. Outcome parameters reported across studies include measures of joint motion, nociception, muscle tone, and performance. Spinal examination procedures include static and dynamic assessments of the quantity and the quality of both active and passive movements. Tiered treatment approaches are recommended to stage the application of various therapies based on ease, cost, and efficacy.

Acupuncture is an inexpensive nonpharmacological modality that has a variety of musculoskeletal, neurologic, and internal medicine applications for the equine practitioner. Common uses include back pain colic, laminitis, laryngeal hemiplegia, and suprascapular neuropathy. Although there is a growing body of literature supporting the use of acupuncture in equids, there remains a need for further robust, double-blinded, placebo-controlled clinical efficacy trials.

Traditional Chinese herbal medicine has been used for the treatment of equine diseases for thousands of years. Clinical studies have found Chinese herbal medicine to be an effective treatment for a variety of equine conditions, and extensive toxicology studies performed on more than 12,000 Chinese herbs provide guidance for safe administration in the horse. Chinese herbal medicine may be used for preventive medicine as well as an integrative or complementary modality for common equine diseases and injuries.

Physiotherapeutic exercises aimed at stimulating motor control, flexibility, and stability are regularly employed in human physical therapy programs. Specifically, the use of such exercises has been shown to reduce both pain and reinjury. Pursuant to the equine patient, several core strengthening exercises and their role in activating deep epaxial musculature to subsequently improve postural motor control and alter thoracolumbar kinematics have been investigated. Both baited and passive exercises offer opportunities to facilitate stretching during dynamic phases and strengthening during static phases of exercise. Blanket recommendations regarding prescription of exercises is not advised, individual patient prescription should be considered in context of handler safety, specific rehabilitation goals, and patient ability to effectively complete the exercise.

 Video content accompanies this article at http://www.vetequine. theclinics.com.

This article provides the equine practitioner with a review of sacroiliac joint pain and dysfunction and outlines the importance of providing a specific prescription for a safe and effective therapeutic exercise program. The continuum of clinical dysfunction associated with the sacroiliac region is presented with prescribed interventions. The intent is to encourage the practitioner to perform a thorough assessment of the sacroiliac joint and the adjacent soft tissues and to use sound clinical reasoning to formulate a therapeutic exercise plan.

VETERINARY CLINICS OF NORTH AMERICA: EQUINE PRACTICE

SERIES OF RELATED INTEREST

Veterinary Clinics of North America: Food Animal Practice
https://www.vetfood.theclinics.com/

THE CLINICS ARE NOW AVAILABLE ONLINE!
Access your subscription at:
www.theclinics.com

Preface

Integrative Medicine: What Is it Good for?

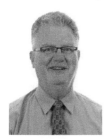

Kevin K. Haussler, DVM, DC, PhD
Editor

It is an honor to be invited to be the guest editor for this issue of *Veterinary Clinics of North America: Equine Practice* that explores some of the modalities that are routinely used within integrative medicine practices. I am acutely aware that after decades of clinical use and continued scientific explorations, the topic of integrative medicine may remain controversial to a certain proportion of equine practitioners. However, a large majority of veterinarians, veterinary students, and horse owners have used many of these techniques to diagnose and manage select musculoskeletal or neurologic disorders in themselves and their equine patients. Personally, I would not be able complete a basic musculoskeletal evaluation without using specific observational skills to assess subtle behavioral changes or proprioceptive deficits or incorporate the requisite soft tissue palpation and joint mobilization techniques without advanced training in manual therapy, acupuncture, and physical rehabilitation. As has been said, "Your treatment is only as good as your diagnosis." The field of integrative medicine has greatly expanded and has become a mainstay within most sports medicine practices, as many horse owners are demanding a more sophisticated approach to the diagnosis and management of subtle performance-limiting issues, and many equine practitioners are frustrated with the limitations of routine diagnostic or treatment options for addressing some of these challenging cases. The sole reliance on pharmaceutics or surgical approaches can only provide a certain level of care, especially for chronic disease processes, vague lameness, or poorly defined performance issues. There are very few horses that can be managed solely on nonsteroidal antiinflammatories (NSAIDs) drugs or corticosteroids for musculoskeletal injuries or sustain prolonged athletic careers without incorporating basic stretching exercises, myofascial work, or physical rehabilitation. Options for providing preventative care or the management of retired or geriatric horses to optimize well-being and quality of life have also been largely supported by incorporating integrative medicine approaches.

Vet Clin Equine 38 (2022) xi–xii
https://doi.org/10.1016/j.cveq.2022.06.002
0749-0739/22/© 2022 Published by Elsevier Inc.

vetequine.theclinics.com

In this issue, readers will learn how to approach clinical cases from a whole-horse perspective and to apply a wide range of appropriate therapies in a staged manner. It is not the intent to review the basic application or mechanisms of action for each individual therapy, which has been reported in many prior publications and can be referenced elsewhere. Our goal is to provide an educated glimpse into the integrative medicine toolbox and to select whatever therapies are available to us that have been shown to be safe and have some level of clinical or scientific evidence of effectiveness for specific disease conditions. General clinical disorders will be approached in a staged or tiered diagnostic or therapeutic approach whereby readily available treatments will be prescribed first and more advanced procedures or treatments with higher costs or risk:benefit ratios will be recommended at later stages of disease development. It is hoped that most clinicians presented with a horse with back pain do not opt for interspinous ligament desmotomy as an initial treatment option, but instead provide a carefully guided progression through several stages of treatment prior to making the final decision to elect for a prescribed surgical procedure. And once surgery has been performed, then the patient is not put immediately back into ridden exercise but is provided an individually tailored rehabilitation program that incorporates a wide range of therapeutic options to restore function, maximize athletic performance, and limit recurrence or comorbidities. The role of proper tack fit and use and an introduction to select rider asymmetries and impairments is also discussed, as these topics are critical for managing the ridden horse but are unfortunately frequently relegated to paraprofessionals, as the human rider is not considered to be within the scope of veterinary medicine. The intent of this issue is to provide an objective foundation on which to base claims of effectiveness and to direct clinical practice efforts.

Kevin K. Haussler, DVM, DC, PhD
Department of Clinical Sciences
Colorado State University
2350 Gillette Drive
1621 Campus Delivery
Fort Collins, CO 80523-1621, USA

E-mail address:
Kevin.Haussler@colostate.edu

Integrative Medicine in Equine Practice

Kevin K. Haussler, DVM, DC, PhD

KEYWORDS

• Horse • Philosophy • Health • Preventative care • Wholistic • Individualized care

KEY POINTS

- There is a growing demand for the use of integrative medicine approaches in equine practice.
- Integrative medicine incorporates all available diagnostic and therapeutic tools to provide the highest level of individualized health care possible.
- Integrative medicine focuses on optimizing the health and wellness of the patient instead of disease processes.

WHAT IS INTEGRATIVE MEDICINE?

Integrative medicine is based on a model of being proactive and promoting health and well-being across an animal's lifetime, rather than being reactive and solely focusing on episodic disease processes.[1] Through individualized care, integrative medicine goes beyond the sole treatment of clinical signs to address all potential underlying causes and effects of an illness. In doing so, the patient's immediate health needs as well as the long-term implications and complex interplay between biological, behavioral, psychosocial, and environmental influences are considered.[2] Integrative medicine strategies also focus on preventive measures and the development of skills for effective self-care.

The term integrative medicine refers to the blending of all aspects of medicine, which includes conventional (eg, pharmaceuticals, surgery), alternative (eg, traditional Chinese medicine, Ayurvedic medicine), and complementary (eg, physical therapy, chiropractic) practices.[3] Additional fields of interest in equine practice may include assessing behavior, providing nutritional recommendations, evaluating tack fit and use, farriery, overseeing training and conditioning programs, and observing horse-rider interactions (**Fig. 1**). Integrative medicine provides the opportunity and supports a willingness to use all appropriate diagnostic and therapeutic approaches whether they originate in conventional, alternative or complementary medicine, and combine

Department of Clinical Sciences, Equine Orthopaedic Research Center, Colorado State University, 2350 Gillette Drive, 1621 Campus Delivery, Fort Collins, CO 80523-1621, USA
E-mail address: Kevin.Haussler@colostate.edu

Vet Clin Equine 38 (2022) 445–453
https://doi.org/10.1016/j.cveq.2022.06.003
0749-0739/22/© 2022 Elsevier Inc. All rights reserved.

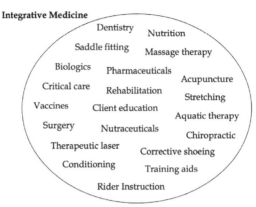

Fig. 1. Illustration of the different tools that might be available to the equine practitioner under the umbrella of integrative medicine.

them so as to have "the best of all worlds" while still maintaining the integrity of each system.[4] The overall goal is to use the most appropriate, safe, effective, and evidence-based modalities available to provide an individualized, whole-body approach to manage disease and promote health.[5]

Practitioners must keep the whole patient in mind and consider how one aspect or part of the body is related to other body regions and how the individual patient interacts with and relates to the external environment and others (ie, human and horse).[6] A common fault in veterinary medicine is to focus attention on a positive diagnostic imaging finding (eg, tarsal osteoarthritis) and to overlook or minimize its influence on other aspects of the body (eg, back pain, ridden exercise). Although corticosteroid injections of the tarsal articulations may resolve the clinical signs of limb lameness, in most cases little to no effort has been made to evaluate any residual or unresolved thoracolumbar pain or stiffness associated with maladaptive compensatory mechanisms. Holistic health care considers the entire spectrum of health from health promotion to health maintenance and injury prevention.[6] Sports medicine and rehabilitative practices have also provided a significant contribution to integrative medicine via diagnostic approaches that focus on evaluating and optimizing function and by providing treatment approaches that emphasize rehabilitation and prescriptive activities that support a return to athletic use and optimized performance. Integrative medicine incorporates a holistic approach to clinical practice that encourages owner involvement with a focus on self-care (ie, home exercises), maintained wellness, optimized function or performance, and disease prevention.[7]{Burton, 2006 #15582}

The term integrative medicine has many contrasting or confusing meanings for different people. The defining principles of veterinary integrative medicine are[2,8]

- The animal owner and practitioner are partners in the healing process
- Health promotion and the illness prevention are of paramount importance
- All factors that influence health, wellness, and disease are taken into consideration
- Care is personalized to best address the owner and the individual patient's unique conditions, needs, and circumstances
- All viable approaches are used to facilitate the body's innate healing responses

- Effective interventions that are safe and less invasive are used whenever possible
- A broad range of diagnostic and therapeutic options are considered that include the physical, behavioral, and environmental aspects that contribute to the disease process and healing
- A team-based approach is encouraged with multidisciplinary specialists collaborating to provide the best diagnostic and effective treatment options possible
- There is an active use of evidence-based medicine principles and available resources across scientific disciplines

BENEFITS OF INTEGRATIVE MEDICINE

In most instances, veterinarians have moved beyond the proverbial medical advice of "Take two aspirin and call me in the morning." Clients expect to receive the best that veterinary medicine has to offer with personalized service, individualized patient care, advanced diagnostics, and safe and effective treatment options. Integrative medicine provides opportunities for assessing pain behavior (eg, ethograms), incorporating chronic pain management strategies, enhanced tissue healing (eg, biological therapies), biomechanical analysis of movement (eg, inertial sensors), tailored rehabilitation programs, and recommendations for injury prevention. Therefore, the diagnostic process is often quite extensive and focused on evaluating the whole-body response to injury or illness. Integrative medicine views health as multidimensional with complex interactions (ie, a system-based approach).[9] Subsequent treatment plans are often tiered to provide gradations of intensity and include therapeutic trials with close monitoring and cost:benefit considerations.

Although conventional veterinary medicine has made substantial advances in diagnostic imaging and the medical and surgical management of equine patients, there remain significant deficits. Early advancements in medicine provided the ability to identify specific etiologic agents (eg, bacteria, fungi, viruses) and then develop effective treatments (ie, antibiotics, antifungals, antivirals). An unintended consequence of this transformation was the reliance on a "find-it-and-fix-it" approach to medical treatment, which emphasizes disease identification and treatment or eradication.[2] Therefore, traditional veterinary medical education and clinical practice have become highly skilled in providing acute care and managing chronic disease processes, with less focus or concurrent training developed in specific methods to prevent injuries, maximize health, or optimize athletic performance. Integrative medicine emphasizes the need to promote health and wellness, rather than waiting for the development of disease.[4] Health promotion and preventative care require a different set of clinical skills and perspectives than is typically provided by a traditional veterinary education or post-graduate training.

Desired traits of a primary health care provider include:[4]
- Knows the patient well and promotes continuity in patient care
- Schedules sufficient time for appointments to address all the owner's questions and concerns
- Able to work effectively with paraprofessionals in a team environment
- Has a working knowledge of traditional, complementary, and alternative therapies
- Able to provide health screening and preventative care
- Has access to a network of reliable referral sources
- Able to direct the owner to the needed critical care
- Acknowledges that the owner and patient's needs may change over time

Within large private practices and educational centers, veterinary care can be fragmented or compartmentalized within sections (eg, dentistry, medicine, surgery). Unfortunately, many surgical patients continue to be discharged without a specific physical therapy assessment or detailed rehabilitation plan with prescribed outcome measures for assessing progress for the return to activities of daily living or sports-specific demands. In horses with poorly defined clinical issues or vague lameness that do not provide the needed information for veterinarians to identify a definitive diagnosis, owners may be told to come back for a recheck appointment when the condition worsens or there are positive findings on subsequent diagnostic evaluations to help to support a pathoanatomical diagnosis. In some instances, diagnostic imaging is used to identify a suspect lesion (eg, cervical osteoarthritis), without any attempt to specifically localize pain, segmental stiffness, or potential functional limitations to determine the perceived clinical relevance of the radiographic findings.

Many integrative medicine practitioners place a strong emphasis on identifying functional changes (eg, pain, stiffness, muscle hypertonicity), which are not readily quantified on routine diagnostic imaging. Therefore, the integrative practitioner is often much more comfortable in dealing with subclinical issues before they become overtly evident on biochemical analysis or routine lameness examination. With the increased clinical use and reliance on inertial sensor systems, the criteria used to definitively diagnose limb lameness are becoming much more nuanced and the gray zone is greatly expanding between subtle motion asymmetries, subclinical gait alterations, and what are judged to be clinically relevant musculoskeletal or neurologic disease processes.

Unfortunately, the management of joint disease in horses continues to rely heavily on intraarticular medications with little focus on extraarticular or contributing factors (eg, altered proprioception, poor motor control, compensatory gait mechanisms). Methods for optimizing performance too often rely on the indiscriminate and routine use of multiple intraarticular corticosteroid injections without clear clinical indications. Although the intent may be to provide individualized treatment; unfortunately, many horses diagnosed with similar disease processes (eg, proximal suspensory desmitis) are often provided quite similar treatment plans without regard for individual differences in the pathogenesis, disease progression, stages of healing, comorbidities, pain or functional adaptations, or athletic disciplines. Finally, assessing appropriate tack fit and use, horse-rider interactions, and rider skills or asymmetries are commonly relegated to paraprofessionals with limited follow-up and little integration or considerations for the concurrent medical or surgical management of individual patients.

Traditional veterinary education is often perceived as monolithic and has significant challenges in updating curricula in response to new medical developments, redefining core competencies, and providing training to emphasize well-being and prevention.[10,11] The valid argument often presented is that there are just too many important topics to teach so there is no extra room within the curriculum to shoehorn in another elective course in veterinary acupuncture or rehabilitation. Therefore, veterinary faculty with training and expertise in integrative medicine approaches have few formal teaching opportunities, and veterinary student education or clinical exposure to nontraditional diagnostic or treatment options is highly varied and is often faculty- or university-dependent.[9] Consequently, postgraduate continuing education is required to provide some basic level of clinical competency in the use of nontraditional medical approaches that are currently deemed requisite skills in most veterinary practices and by most horse owners or trainers.

Equine practitioners that incorporate acupuncture methods into their diagnostic and treatment regimens primarily focus on musculoskeletal issues; however, there is evidence for treating gastrointestinal, reproductive, respiratory, and neurologic disorders.[12] Acupuncture can provide valuable insights into the diagnosis and effective management of chronic pain, where few other options may exist.[13,14] Physical therapy approaches provide unique insights into assessing neuromusculoskeletal function that are mostly lacking in veterinary medicine.[15] Although there is little scientific evidence for the specific application (eg, dosage) and clinical efficacy of many of the therapeutic exercises or physical modalities in horses, most rehabilitation recommendations are based on clinical experience and extrapolation from human studies.[16–18] From a manual therapy perspective, significant contributions have been made in the diagnosis of axial skeleton issues by incorporating basic soft tissue and osseous palpation techniques and by assessing segmental joint motion.[19,20] From a treatment perspective, manual therapies are often the primary means of managing myofascial pain and joint stiffness in the equine athlete.[21–23] Integrative medicine has also provided the much-needed perspectives and opportunities for providing humane palliative care for horses with chronic, progressive, or end-stage disease.[24,25]

WHAT IS AN INTEGRATIVE PRACTICE?

Several models that incorporate integrative medicine practices have been described in human medicine.[8,26] Similar approaches have been used in equine practice, but many do not fully embrace the true intention or full benefits of integrative medicine. The philosophy of many of our teaching institutions continues to base their curricula and clinical activities on the belief that the best possible care is provided by conventional medicine and that integrative medicine is an inferior treatment option (eg, use of NSAIDS vs cryotherapy for acute soft tissue inflammation). At the other extreme, integrative medicine may be perceived as a superior treatment option based on the assumption that there are limited or no specific treatment options available by using conventional medicine approaches (eg, managing neck stiffness with baited carrot stretches or spinal mobilization vs no treatment considered or provided). An intermediary approach might assume that both conventional and integrative treatments are similar in safety and effectiveness, therefore treatment options might be based on the owner or practitioner's preference (eg, generalized muscle hypertonicity treated with muscle relaxants vs myofascial work or acupuncture). However, the best philosophy or true approach of integrative medicine is to use a combination of all diagnostic and treatment options available with equal regard for their specific indications, safety, and clinical efficacy (eg, arthroscopic surgery combined with postoperative rehabilitation).[27]

The selected treatment plan should include the following considerations:[5]
- Is based on the best available evidence to support its clinical use and effectiveness
- Has a favorable risk:benefit ratio compared with other treatment options for the same condition
- Is based on a reasonable expectation that the applied therapy will result in a favorable patient outcome, which includes preventive practices
- Includes close monitoring with objective outcome measures to assess clinical responses
- Is based on the expectation that a greater benefit will be achieved than that which can be expected with no treatment
- Includes the personal preferences of both the owner and practitioner
- Does not delay or preclude any other necessary or more effective evidence-based treatment (eg, the need for surgery in emergency situations)

The long-standing driver for providing integrative health care has been and continues to be client demand.[4] It is uncommon that a practitioner is entirely self-motivated to pursue postgraduate educational programs, accumulate increased personal debt, and take substantial time away from family and clinical duties just for the sake of learning a new therapeutic modality. Fortunately for the veterinary profession, a select group of practitioners have made the required personal sacrifices and have pushed for the development and integration of nontraditional approaches into most equine practices. Owing to the efforts of these individuals, integrative medicine is now increasingly demanded by horse owners and trainers and more commonly accepted by most practitioners, equine practices, and educational institutions.

MODELS OF INTEGRATIVE CARE

The continued misguided advice of stating that "The treatment may help but it can't do any harm" is inappropriate and reflects the obvious lack of awareness of the specific indications or effectiveness of a stated modality. A better and more informed approach would be to state that you do not know the specific indications or effectiveness of a modality (eg, massage therapy), but that you can refer the owner to someone who has more training and experience in that specific modality. The preferred or more proactive approach might be that the practitioner themselves conduct a literature review into a specific issue or participate in continuing education programs, which would then allow them to provide an educated and informed response based on the most up-to-date level of scientific evidence available.

Productive interprofessional collaborations are an essential component to the effective delivery of integrative medicine services.[28] This is especially true for within large multi-practitioner clinics or university-settings but needs to be equally so for private practitioners that are called upon to provide referral services. The broad offerings of integrative medicine are best provided by a team of experts (ie, multidisciplinary approach) instead of the sole reliance on a single individual that is tasked with providing all the required integrative services (eg, acupuncture, chiropractic, physical therapy) within a practice. Although this approach may seem to be the most cost-effective and efficient, it often does not provide the needed depth or breadth of specialized care that most patients require for managing chronic disease processes or for optimizing health.

PATIENT-CENTERED CARE

Integrative medicine practitioners often place a high value on establishing strong interpersonal relationships with their clients, which is based on trust, respect, and includes a personal commitment to devoting the needed time and resources to fully understand the individual client's needs and desires. Human medicine has a long historical record of providing health care delivery from a paternalistic perspective, where a doctor's opinions or recommendations often supersede or do not take into consideration the patient's concerns or desires. It seems that veterinary medicine has been more nibble or nuanced in its approach to health care as the owner serves as an critical intermediary in the veterinary-client-patient relationship. As owner's may often place the needs of their pets or horses above their own health care needs, veterinarians have been able to provide patient-centered care more readily, which is a fundamental component of practicing integrative veterinary medicine.[4] Increased competition between veterinary practices, reduced reliance on third-party payers (ie, health care insurance), and the need for a high compliance rate may also play significant roles in considering the horse owner's financial capabilities and personal needs or desires in recommending referral for advanced diagnostic imaging or designing comprehensive treatment plans. In human medicine, patient-centered care has been shown to improve patient and practitioner satisfaction, lead to better clinical outcomes, and lower malpractice rates.[4] With continued scientific advancements, a larger number of diagnostic and therapeutic options are now available. However, with the advent of the Internet, veterinarians are often placed in the position of attempting to provide the best possible medical care while also trying to guide the owner (or themselves) through the never-ending deluge of confusing or outright misleading medical information or the latest and greatest "technological innovations" based solely on a manufacturer's reported claims of effectiveness. A heighted sense of diligence and rigor is required to evaluate the reported safety and efficacy of the never-ending expansion of purported therapies to determine if they may provide a useful tool to add to the equine practitioner's tool bag of integrative medicine.

CLINICS CARE POINTS

- Step back and observe the entire patient and the surrounding environment. Pay attention to subtle behavioral changes and listen closely to owner or trainer comments and observations.

- Do not limit your examination and treatment only toward the presenting complaint.

- Be passionately curious and always ask why. Why did the horse injury that specific limb and not any another limb? What other contributing factors might influence tissue healing?

- Remember to treat the patient and not the diagnostic imaging findings.

- There is usually more than one way to manage a disease process. Use the safest and most effective treatment possible.

- You did not learn everything that you needed in veterinary school to be an effective practitioner. Ask for help when needed.

- A team approach provides the opportunity for additional opinions and diverse insights that are often required for long-term, comprehensive care.

- An educated owner is the best client that you can ask for.

DISCLOSURE

The author has nothing to disclose.

REFERENCES

1. Hermanson S, Pujari A, Williams B, et al. Successes and challenges of implementing an integrative medicine practice in an allopathic medical center. Healthc (Amst) 2021;9(2):100457.
2. Institute of Medicine. Integrative medicine and the health of the public: a summary of the February 2009 summit. Washington, DC: The National Academies Press; 2009.
3. Gellis JE. Complementary, alternative, and integrative therapies (CAIT). In: Yong RJ, Nguyen M, Nelson E, et al, editors. Pain medicine: an essential review. Cham: Springer International Publishing; 2017. p. 419–27.
4. Maizes V, Rakel D, Niemiec C. Integrative medicine and patient-centered care. Explore (NY) 2009;5(5):277–89.
5. Kotsirilos V, Cohen M, Hassed D, et al. Best practice for integrative medicine in Australian medical practice. Adv Integr Med 2014;1:69–84. https://doi.org/10.

1016/j.aimed.2013.12.001. Australasian Integrative Medicine Association Position Paper. Elsevier Ltd.

6. Xu Y. Complementary and alternative therapies as philosophy and modalities: implications for nursing practice, education, and research. Home Health Care Management Pract 2004;16(6):534–7.

7. Riley DS, Anderson R, Blair JC, et al. The Academy of Integrative Health and Medicine and the Evolution of Integrative Medicine Practice, Education, and Fellowships. Integr Med (Encinitas) 2016;15(1):38–41.

8. Hu X-Y, Lorenc A, Kemper K, et al. Defining integrative medicine in narrative and systematic reviews: A suggested checklist for reporting. Eur J Integr Med 2015; 7(1):76–84.

9. Willison KD. Advancing integrative medicine through interprofessional education. Health Sociol Rev 2008;17(4):342–52.

10. Memon MA, Shmalberg J, Adair HS 3rd, et al. Integrative veterinary medical education and consensus guidelines for an integrative veterinary medicine curriculum within veterinary colleges. Open Vet J 2016;6(1):44–56.

11. Memon MA, Shmalberg JW, Xie H. Survey of integrative veterinary medicine training in AVMA-Accredited veterinary colleges. J Vet Med Educ 2021;48(3): 289–94.

12. Shmalberg J, Xie H, Memon MA. Horses referred to a teaching hospital exclusively for acupuncture and herbs: a three-year retrospective analysis. J Acupuncture Meridian Stud 2019;12(5):145–50.

13. Cantwell SL. Traditional Chinese veterinary medicine: the mechanism and management of acupuncture for chronic pain. Top Companion Anim *Med* 2010; 25(1):53–8.

14. Faramarzi B, Lee D, May K, et al. Response to acupuncture treatment in horses with chronic laminitis. Can Vet J 2017;58(8):823–7.

15. Blanpied PR, Gross AR, Elliott JM, et al. Neck pain: revision 2017. J Orthop Sports Phys Ther 2017;47(7):A1–83.

16. Nankervis KJ, Launder EJ, Murray RC. The use of treadmills within the rehabilitation of horses. J Equine Vet Sci 2017;53:108–15.

17. Clayton HM. Core training and rehabilitation in horses. Vet Clin North Am Equine Pract 2016;32(1):49–71.

18. Haussler KK, King MR, Peck K, et al. The development of safe and effective rehabilitation protocols for horses. Equine Vet Educ 2021;33(3):143–51.

19. Haussler KK. Joint mobilization and manipulation for the equine athlete. Vet Clin North Am Equine Pract 2016;32(1):87–101.

20. Bowen AG, Goff LM, McGowan CM. Investigation of myofascial trigger points in equine pectoral muscles and girth-aversion behavior. J Equine Vet Sci 2017;48: 154–60.e1.

21. Kędzierski W, Janczarek I, Stachurska A, et al. Comparison of effects of different relaxing massage frequencies and different music hours on reducing stress level in race horses. J Equine Vet Sci 2017;53:100–7.

22. Kowalik S, Janczarek I, Kędzierski W, et al. The effect of relaxing massage on heart rate and heart rate variability in purebred Arabian racehorses. Anim Sci J 2017;88(4):669–77.

23. Hill C, Crook T. The relationship between massage to the equine caudal hindlimb muscles and hindlimb protraction. Equine Vet J 2010;42(s38):683–7.

24. Selter F, Persson K, Risse J, et al. Dying like a dog: the convergence of concepts of a good death in human and veterinary medicine. Med Health Care Philos 2022; 25(1):73–86.

25. Hurn S, Badman-King A. Care as an alternative to euthanasia? reconceptualizing veterinary palliative and end-of-life care. Med Anthropol Q 2019;33(1):138–55.
26. Patterson C, Arthur HM. A model for implementing integrative practice in health care agencies. Integr Med Insights 2008;3:13–9.
27. Shmalberg J, Memon MA. A retrospective analysis of 5,195 patient treatment sessions in an integrative veterinary medicine service: patient characteristics, presenting complaints, and therapeutic interventions. Vet Med Int 2015;2015: 983621.
28. Chung VCH, Ma PHX, Hong LC, et al. Organizational determinants of interprofessional collaboration in integrative health care: systematic review of qualitative studies. PLoS One 2012;7(11):e50022.

Integrative Philosophy
Case Management

Steve Adair, MS, DVM

KEYWORDS

- Integrative medicine • Complementary medicine • Case management
- Pain management • Tissue healing • Mental health

KEY POINTS

- Integrative philosophy pertains to the thoughtful consideration and combination of conventional Western medicine with complementary medicine.
- The goal of integrative medicine is to improve the health of the patient in a more holistic manner.
- The equine practitioner is the most qualified professional to address the individual patient's needs and to coordinate care with the help of a team of professionals.

INTRODUCTION

According to the National Center for Complementary and Integrative Health, integrative medicine brings conventional and complementary approaches together in a coordinated way to provide high-quality scientific evidence of safety and effectiveness of multimodal interventions, such as conventional approaches (eg, medication, physical rehabilitation, and surgery) and complementary approaches (eg, acupuncture, massage, nutrition, and chiropractic) in various combinations.[1,2] Integrative case management aims for coordinated care among different providers by bringing conventional and complementary approaches together to care for the whole individual.[2]

The American Veterinary Medical Association (AVMA) Model Practice Act considers complementary, alternative, and integrative therapies as a heterogeneous group of preventive, diagnostic, and therapeutic philosophies and practices that are not considered part of conventional (Western) medicine as practiced by most veterinarians and veterinary technicians or technologists.[3] These therapies include, but are not limited to, veterinary acupuncture, acutherapy, and acupressure; veterinary homeopathy; veterinary manual or manipulative therapy (ie, therapies based on techniques practiced in osteopathy and chiropractic); veterinary nutraceutical therapy; and veterinary phytotherapy.[4] The AVMA believes that all aspects of veterinary medicine should

Department of Large Animal Clinical Science, University of Tennessee, College of Veterinary Medicine, 2407 River Drive, Knoxville, TN 37996-4545, USA
E-mail address: sadair@utk.edu

Vet Clin Equine 38 (2022) 455–461
https://doi.org/10.1016/j.cveq.2022.06.004
0749-0739/22/© 2022 Elsevier Inc. All rights reserved.
vetequine.theclinics.com

be held to the same standards, including complementary, alternative, and integrative veterinary medicine, nontraditional or other novel approaches.[5]

Why Do Clients Seek Integrative Care?

It is important to understand why clients seek an integrative care approach to their horse's health. Many of their reasons are like what has been found in human medicine. According to Powell,[1] the following are reasons provided for seeking integrative approaches in human medicine:

- Studies show that individuals turn to these integrative medicine approaches because they consider them to be more aligned with their values, beliefs, and philosophies about health than a strictly conventional medical approach.
- Some patients prefer the customized, personal care that comes with integrative medicine's whole-person perspective.
- Some believe it is logical to incorporate health strategies into their lives from the widest array of proven approaches possible.
- Studies have been conducted that demonstrate that the patients who participate in integrative medicine programs realize more profound health benefits than those who do not.
- The integrative medicine model recognizes the critical role the practitioner–patient relationship plays in a patient's overall health care experience.

Many of these reasons also apply to our veterinary–client–patient relationship. Although the horse cannot make the decision as to their preferred health care, their owners certainly can. Other factors that enter into the decision are related to the financial aspect of their horse's care, dissatisfaction with the current level of care, or the lack of response to conventional medicine.

Team-Based Approach

For the equine practitioner, it is important to know what complementary therapies exist, their basic mechanisms of action, clinical indications, potential adverse effects, and how to best integrate them into traditional practice. A suggested model for an integrative system is based on the team-based care with the veterinarian serving as the case manager.[6] The veterinarian is often the person who knows the patient the best, is able to oversee the patient's needs, and coordinates care with the help of a team of professionals. The equine practitioner must strive to identify the appropriate diagnosis and decide on the appropriate therapy. The veterinarian must be willing and able to either provide the needed service or to coordinate its delivery with a team of qualified professionals. Together, the team can meet all the health needs of the individual patient. For the veterinarian to be a team leader, they must be familiar with the plethora of modalities and interventions available and what evidenced-based knowledge exists which documents treatment efficacy for a particular clinical issue. Complementary therapies may include acupuncture, veterinary manipulative therapy, physical rehabilitation, photobiomodulation, therapeutic exercises, stretching, massage, integrative nutrition, and botanic medicine to name a few.[7–10] Unfortunately, there is a lack of well-controlled studies that document efficacy of most complementary therapies used in horses, thus the practitioner must rely on personal experience and scientific evidence that might be available in other species.[10] It is encouraging that more research is being done and integrative medicine is being incorporated into the veterinary educational system.[7,9]

As a team leader and the case manager, the equine practitioner must be willing to take more of a holistic approach to their patient's care, which includes the areas of pain management, tissue healing, and mental health. Pain management is typically the primary lameness or rehabilitation issue to address in most equine patients. Unfortunately, conventional practice still has a limited armamentarium for managing chronic pain syndromes in horses. Supporting the tissue healing process via biological therapies, controlled exercise, or physical modalities is another important aspect of integrative medicine. When considering long-term management and activity modifications required for the effective treatment of severe or recurrent injuries, the behavioral aspects and mental health of the equine patient are of paramount importance. The difference between a well-balanced, cooperative patient and one that is not can be the difference between treatment success and failure.

Pain Management

To address pain, the equine practitioner must be able to recognize and quantify the level of pain. There are many methods available that are both subjective and objective. Physiologic and observational parameters are often used but more recently more quantifiable methods have been developed. Inertial sensor systems are now available to quantify the degree of gait asymmetry that often relates to lameness.[11] Recently, pain ethograms have been developed[12,13] for the horse in an attempt to decrease the subjective nature of observation. By using these monitoring tools, the equine practitioner can quantifiably measure pain and response to treatment. This allows for adjustment of the therapeutic plan, if indicated.

To address pain from a non-pharmacological perceptive, the equine practitioner often has many safe and effective options to consider. Acupuncture has been shown to be a safe therapy with minimal side effects to address pain in horses.[14] Local, spinal, and brain effects of acupuncture involve enhanced release of pain-relieving endogenous substances and inhibiting the release of pain-inducing substances.[15] Manual therapies are directed toward relieving sensory, neuromuscular, and mechanical abnormalities.[16] Aquatic therapy may aid in relief of musculoskeletal pain due to buoyancy, hydrostatic pressure, and thermal effects.[16–18] Cryotherapy has been shown to decrease pain and reduce swelling and inflammation.[19] There are many different methods for the application of cold in the horse.[20–22] Photobiomodulation or low-level laser therapy may also have both analgesic and anti-inflammatory effects.[23–25] Transelectrical nerve stimulation is used in humans for the treatment of chronic pain.[26–28] However, its use in the horse for effective pain management has yet to be confirmed. Extracorporeal shockwave therapy has been shown to transiently reduce pain in horses.[29,30] Therapeutic ultrasound may also have analgesic effect due to its thermal effects causing vasodilation.[16]

Tissue Healing

Many of the modalities or interventions presented above may also help to support and improve tissue healing. Manual therapies such as massage, myofascial release, or trigger point therapy may aid in postexercise recovery, pain reduction, and improved range of motion.[31] Similarly, stretching may decrease tissue scarring and improve range of motion and flexibility post-injury.[32] Both therapeutic ultrasound and extracorporeal shockwave therapy have an effect at both the tissue and cellular level that may aid in tissue healing.[26,33,34] Photobiomodulation has been shown to promote healing of soft tissue injuries and wounds.[35–37] Hyperbaric oxygen therapy is a promising therapy for tissue healing. Its potential is well-documented in humans but is controversial in horses as there are conflicting reports of efficacy.[38–41]

Mental Health

Often, we focus on the physical condition of our patient and neglect the behavioral or mental aspects. Specific focus on a clinical issue (ie, tunnel vision) often affects our management of a case. To effectively manage disease or injury, the practitioner must consider the entire horse which is one of the foundations of integrative medicine. There are multiple factors that can affect a horse's mental status. Smith and colleagues[42] developed the "BICEPS" concept that focuses on the mental and emotional aspect of therapy and rehabilitation. BICEPS is an acronym for six different categories related to the mental status of the horse that include: boredom, isolation, confinement, environment, pain, and staff. Each of these categories should be individually addressed by using different interventions to improve the horse's overall mental status. Boredom and isolation often contribute to the development of stereotypic behaviors.[42,43] Boredom may be counteracted in the stall-confined patient by using different objects in the stall that engages the horse mentally. An example would be a ball hay feeder that the horse must push around the stall to be able to access the hay. If at all possible, the horse should be taken out of the stall several times a day and allowed controlled movement. To counteract isolation, another horse can be placed in the stall next to or across from the patient. Horses are social animals and having companions within sight often help them to remain mentally stable. An articulated brace may be used to counteract overloading of the injured structures in horses with suspensory apparatus or flexor tendon injuries. A clean environment is a must. Frequent cleaning of the stall is important to prevent skin irritations and decrease odors. A well-ventilated barn is also important to decrease the incidence of respiratory issues. The importance of pain management and the interventions and modalities that may be used has been discussed above. Last, it is important to have well-trained staff that understand the nuances of equine behavior, can recognize when a horse's behavior is changing, and are comfortable handling horses with a variety of perceived personality types.

SUMMARY

The equine practitioner is the most qualified person to take on the role of a team leader or case manager and to facilitate all aspects of patient care provided by many different individuals. In this capacity, the equine practitioner must either provide the complementary care themselves or be receptive to allowing another professional or paraprofessional to provide those services, as deemed appropriate.

CLINICS CARE POINTS

- The Equine Veterinarian should be the "Case Manager" that cooridinates patient care.
- The Equine Veterinarian does not need to provide complimentary therapy but should be familiar with the complimentary approaches recommended.
- The Equine Veternarian should do frequent re-evaluations to determine if the complimantary therapy is providing added benefit.

CONFLICTS OF INTEREST

None.

REFERENCES

1. Powell SK. Integrative Medicine and Case Management. Prof Case Management 2016;21:111–3.
2. Anon. Complementary, Alternative, or Integrative Health: What's In a Name? NCCIH. Available at: https://www.nccih.nih.gov/health/complementary-alternative-or-integrative-health-whats-in-a-name. Accessed January 26, 2022.
3. Anon. Model Veterinary Practice Act. Am Vet Med Assoc.. Available at: https://www.avma.org/resources-tools/avma-policies/model-veterinary-practice-act. Accessed May 24, 2022.
4. Meacham N. 2019 model veterinary practice act. 2019. Available at: https://www.avma.org/sites/default/files/2021-01/model-veterinary-practice-act.pdf.
5. Complementary Anon. alternative, and integrative veterinary medicine. Am Vet Med Assoc. Available at: https://www.avma.org/resources-tools/avma-policies/complementary-alternative-and-integrative-veterinary-medicine. Accessed September 30, 2020.
6. Maizes V, Rakel D, Niemiec C. Integrative Medicine and Patient-Centered Care. EXPLORE 2009;5:277–89.
7. Memon MA, Shmalberg J, Adair HS III, et al. Integrative veterinary medical education and consensus guidelines for an integrative veterinary medicine curriculum within veterinary colleges. Open Vet J 2016;6:44–56.
8. Memon MA, Shmalberg JW, Xie H. Survey of Integrative Veterinary Medicine Training in AVMA-Accredited Veterinary Colleges. J Vet Med Educ 2021;48:289–94.
9. Devine S. Integrative equine sports medicine. Vet Ireland J 2018;8:661–3.
10. Haussler K. Current Status of Integrative Medicine Techniques Used in Equine Practice. J Equine Vet Sci 2009;29:639–41.
11. Keegan KG. Evidence-based lameness detection and quantification. Vet Clin North Am Equine Pract 2007;23:403–23.
12. Torcivia C, McDonnell S. Equine Discomfort Ethogram. Animals 2021;11:580.
13. Dyson S, Berger J, Ellis AD, et al. Development of an ethogram for a pain scoring system in ridden horses and its application to determine the presence of musculoskeletal pain. J Vet Behav 2018;23:47–57.
14. le Jeune S, Henneman K, May K. Acupuncture and Equine Rehabilitation. Vet Clin North Am Equine Pract 2016;32:73–85.
15. Dewey C, Xie H. The scientific basis of acupuncture for veterinary pain management: a review based on relevant literature from the last two decades. Open Vet J 2021;11:203.
16. Daglish J, Mama KR. Pain: Its Diagnosis and Management in the Rehabilitation of Horses. Vet Clin North Am Equine Pract 2016;32:13–29.
17. King M. Principles and application of hydrotherapy for equine athletes. Vet Clin North Am Equine Pract 2016;32(1):115–26.
18. King MR, Haussler KK, Kawcak CE, et al. Mechanisms of aquatic therapy and its potential use in managing equine osteoarthritis. Equine Vet Education 2013;25:204–9.
19. Belanger A-Y. Cryotherapy. In: Therapeutic electrophysical agents - evidence behind practice. 2nd edition. Philadelphia, PA: Lippincott Williams & Wilkens; 2010. p. 121–49.
20. van Eps AW, Walters LJ, Baldwin GI, et al. Distal limb cryotherapy for the prevention of acute laminitis. Clin Tech Equine Pract 2004;3:64–70.
21. van Eps AW, Orsini JA. A comparison of seven methods for continuous therapeutic cooling of the equine digit. Equine Vet J 2016;48:120–4.

22. Hunt ER. Response of twenty-seven horses with lower leg injuries to cold spa bath hydrotherapy. J Equine Vet Sci 2001;21:188–93.

23. Ahmed W, Elbrønd VS, Harrison AP, et al. An investigation into the short-term effects of photobiomodulation on the mechanical nociceptive thresholds of M. longissimus and M. gluteus medius, in relation to muscle firing rate in horses at three different gaits. J Equine Vet Sci 2020;98:103363.

24. Haussler KK, Manchon PT, Donnell JR, et al. Effects of low-level laser therapy and chiropractic care on back pain in quarter horses. J Equine Vet Sci 2020;86: 102891.

25. Hochman L. Photobiomodulation therapy in veterinary medicine: a review. Topics in companion animal medicine. 2018. Available at: https://linkinghub.elsevier.com/retrieve/pii/S1938973618300011. Accessed July 12, 2018.

26. Baxter GD, McDonough SM. Principles of electrotherapy in veterinary physiotherapy. In: Animal physiotherapy: assessment, treatment and rehabilitation of animals. Ames, IA: Blackwell Publishing; 2007. p. 177–86.

27. Belanger A-Y. Transcutaneous electrical nerve stimulation therapy. In: Therapeutic electrophysical agents - evidence behind practice. Philadelphia, PA: Lippincott Williams & Wilkens; 2010. p. 277–305.

28. Johnson M. Transcutaneous electrical nerve stimulation: review of effectiveness. Nurs Stand 2014;28:44–53.

29. Dahlberg JA, McClure SR, Evans RB, et al. Force platform evaluation of lameness severity following extracorporeal shock wave therapy in horses with unilateral forelimb lameness. J Am Vet Med Assoc 2006;229:100–3.

30. McClure SR, Sonea IM, Evans RB, et al. Evaluation of analgesia resulting from extracorporeal shock wave therapy and radial pressure wave therapy in the limbs of horses and sheep. Am J Vet Res 2005;66:1702–8.

31. Scott M, Swenson LA. Evaluating the benefits of equine massage therapy: a review of the evidence and current practices. J Equine Vet Sci 2009;29:687–97.

32. Frick A. Stretching exercises for horses: are they effective? J Equine Vet Sci 2010; 30:50–9.

33. Yocom AF, Bass LD. Review of the application and efficacy of extracorporeal shockwave therapy in equine tendon and ligament injuries. Equine Vet Educ 2019;31:271–7.

34. Yilmaz V, Karadas O, Dandinoglu T, et al. Efficacy of extracorporeal shockwave therapy and low-intensity pulsed ultrasound in a rat knee osteoarthritis model: A randomized controlled trial. Eur J Rheumatol 2017;4:104–8.

35. Hoisang S, Kampa N, Seesupa S, et al. Assessment of wound area reduction on chronic wounds in dogs with photobiomodulation therapy: a randomized controlled clinical trial. Vet World 2021;14(8):2251–9.

36. Pluim M, Martens A, Vanderperren K, et al. Short- and long term follow-up of 150 sports horses diagnosed with tendinopathy or desmopathy by ultrasonographic examination and treated with high-power laser therapy. Res Vet Sci 2018;119: 232–8.

37. Pluim M, Heier A, Plomp S, et al. Histological tissue healing following high-power laser treatment in a model of suspensory ligament branch injury. Equine Vet J. Available at: https://onlinelibrary.wiley.com/doi/abs/10.1111/evj.13556. Accessed January 24, 2022.

38. Baumwart CA, Doherty TJ, Schumacher J, et al. Effects of hyperbaric oxygen treatment on horses with experimentally induced endotoxemia. Am J Vet Res 2011;72:1266–75.

39. Górski K, Stefanik E, Bereznowski A, et al. Application of hyperbaric oxygen therapy (HBOT) as a healing aid after extraction of incisors in the equine odontoclastic tooth resorption and hypercementosis syndrome. Vet Sci 2022;9:30.
40. Holder TEC, Schumacher J, Donnell RL, et al. Effects of hyperbaric oxygen on full-thickness meshed sheet skin grafts applied to fresh and granulating wounds in horses. Am J Vet Res 2008;69:144–7.
41. Barnes RC. Point: Hyperbaric Oxygen Is Beneficial for Diabetic Foot Wounds. Clin Infect Dis 2006;43:188–92.
42. Smith C, Miller RM, Parelli P. Psychological aspects of rehabilitation. In: Rehabilitating the athletic horse. Hauppauge, NY: Nova Science Publishers, Inc.; 2013. p. 179–201.
43. Prescott K. Optimising the welfare of equids on box rest: thinking outside the box. UK-Vet Equine 2021;5:122–8.

Optimizing Health – Integrative Medicine & Poor Performance

Kimberly Henneman, DVM, Diplomate ACVSMR (Equine, Canine), CVA (IVAS), CVC (AVCA)

KEYWORDS

- Acupuncture • Traditional Asian (Chinese) veterinary medicine • Manual therapy
- Chiropractic • Osteopathy • Homeopathy • Herbal medicine • Ayurvedic medicine

KEY POINTS

- Poor performance in the horse may encompass a variety of hard-to-diagnose causes involving multiple organ systems.
- The application of integrative therapies for poor performance gives veterinary practitioners extra tools for diagnosis and treatment.
- Maximizing the utilization of various integrative modalities in practice involves additional professional training and understanding of modality philosophies.

Abbreviations	
TCVM	Traditional Chinese Veterinary Medicine

INTRODUCTION

Poor performance problems, exercise intolerance, and horses that are "just not quite right" are common reasons why equine veterinarians are asked to examine and treat many equine patients. However, most of the equine literature is unable to specifically define poor performance and the clinical presentations encompass a wide and confusing variety of clinical signs. Pursuing causes for the varied list of clinical signs that are often present in horses being evaluated for "poor performance" involves combining flexible thinking with thorough physical evaluations. Besides the pulmonary and cardiovascular organ systems that can affect stamina and energy, just considering clinical musculoskeletal causes alone can present what can seem to the clinician as an infinite variety of potential causes, yet integrative therapies combined with conventional medicine can help the clinician with diagnosis and treatment.

Integrative therapies as used today refer to a varied group of nonconventional therapies such as Traditional Asian (Chinese) Medicine, Medical acupuncture, Ayurvedic

Animal Health VIPS, 3070 W. Rasmussen Road Suite 80, Park City, UT 84098, USA
E-mail address: ahooffice@aol.com

Vet Clin Equine 38 (2022) 463–474
https://doi.org/10.1016/j.cveq.2022.08.001
0749-0739/22/© 2022 Elsevier Inc. All rights reserved.

Medicine, chiropractic, osteopathy, physical rehabilitation, herbal medicine or phyto-therapy, homeopathy, and nutraceuticals. They have been growing in both popular and clinical use throughout the international equine world, despite many modalities still not quite reaching the current standards of evidence-based efficacy and safety research.[1-5] While some of these modalities do lack more modern scientific evaluations, most integrative therapies have decades, if not centuries and millennia, of wide clinical usage in multiple species by trained practitioners using long-established, consistent and defined protocols. Despite many modalities initially being used without adequate research scrutiny, the body of evidence for most of the various modalities continues to grow rapidly as technology finally catches up with years of clinical expertise and usage. To put it in perspective, acupuncture was in use for more than 2000 years before the endorphin receptor was discovered in 1973, providing the first viable explanation for acupuncture responses. Now, acupuncture research has shown neurologic, endocrine, vascular, lymphatic, fascial, and musculoskeletal mechanisms of action. Research on many other modalities also continues to increase.

MAKING THE SHIFT IN MEDICAL PERSPECTIVE

The modern Western medical approach to solving disease is to break complex biolog-ical problems into clinical signs compartmentalized via body systems, then going through accepted algorithms designed to isolate a dysfunction; this is often referred to as the reductionist method. Even if multiple organs could be involved, they are iso-lated and treated as separate and mostly unrelated problems. In contrast, most inte-grative modalities, especially Traditional Chinese (Asian) Medicine, Indian Ayurveda, Western European Classical Homeopathy, and Chiropractic or Osteopathy view the body as a totally integrated whole. This body-global approach, present as the founda-tion in many integrative techniques, has resulted in the development of unique, and sometimes very different, physiologic and pathophysiologic patterning approaches to body systems and their relationships in both health and disease.

When looking at integrative modalities from different cultures with different technolo-gies which evolved over centuries and millennia, it is important for today's practitioners to understand and respect the foundational distinctions between a particular modality and modern Western medicine. The organization of a modality's patterns of clinical signs may be different—not bad, not good, just different. Flexibility in thinking between ap-proaches allows a clinician to see where certain clinical sign patterns may overlap (despite having different names), and how one pattern may provide insight into the level of health or disease that a more conventional pattern may miss. This is the strength of adding integrative therapies to modern medicine when attempting to deal with chal-lenging or vague complaints. It also means that the clinician wanting to use these thera-pies should be willing to learn the language of each modality which has evolved over time due to the clinical expertise and observations of the practitioners who have gone before.

INTEGRATIVE THERAPY MODALITIES IN HEALTH AND PERFORMANCE

A conventionally trained practitioner adding an integrative modality to their training does not throw away the knowledge gleaned through veterinary school and years of practice experience. Rather, adding the modality training to a solid medical foundation helps to provide context for its usage. Because of the differences in how medical pat-terns are described for each modality, proper education followed by practice mentor-ship and usage practice can help a clinician's expertise with the tool. Understanding how an integrative modality is practiced can make clinicians aware of when a partic-ular modality provides information that can fill in a missing examination or diagnostic piece that modern Western medicine may not recognize. The more medical tools a practitioner has, the more information is acquired. More data can help clinicians classify outliers into a modality's descriptive hierarchy, thus possibly providing other options for treatment. Clinical signs that once were meaningless and often ignored in Western medical disease patterns, now take on value and importance within the dysfunction patterning of an integrative modality's approach.

Another benefit of adding integrative therapies is the ability to offer clients more options for treatment. Not only can this help avert a feeling of helplessness on the part of the veterinarian, but it can help build client bonds, especially with outlier cases. The veterinarian is at least trying to do something if other treatment options are unavailable to the client. Having additional tools such as chiropractic or osteopathy, acupuncture & herbs (especially based on Traditional precepts), rehabilitation, or manual therapy, allows a veterinary practitioner to still feel and be useful in the field when a client cannot afford certain surgical or medical interventions, the horse is unable to trailer to a facility offering advanced care, or there isn't an advanced care facility in the area.

WHY ADD INTEGRATIVE THERAPIES IN POOR PERFORMANCE CASES?

Poor performance problems can be caused by one or more issues involving one or multiple body systems. As Hinchcliff states, "Maximal performance involves the coordinated optimal functioning of almost all body systems."[6] Any single disturbance in the complex functioning of heart, lungs, muscles, blood vessels, energy metabolism, hormonal signaling, tendons, ligaments, and fascia has the potential of causing deviations from normal performance and even from optimal health. The stacking of multiple dysfunctions makes for even more complicated health and performance problems. Some deviations are present in obvious ways, but most tend to be more subtle where recognition may be subject to the observational skills of the owner and veterinarian.

Western medical technology excels in finding and diagnosing measurable and structural changes, for example, tendon cross-sectional area, red blood cell count, and histopathology. But, many causes of lethargy, fatigue, or low-grade gait abnormalities can come from subtle functional problems rather than those more easily detectable. Many performance problems are slowly progressive and usually don't start as a sudden loss in the structural integrity of a particular anatomic part, as equine veterinarians with those early twinges, stiffnesses, and sore muscles can attest to. Therefore, determining the causes of poor performance or just "being off" with conventional tools can be challenging for the equine clinician.

Western medicine-trained practitioners should realize that knowing the mechanics or *SCIENCE* of how these therapies are thought to work is not enough for fully successful integration into practice. The philosophies of many integrative modalities can be very different from more modern medical perspectives. Therefore, to incorporate an integrative approach effectively with a more conventional one, an interested clinician must also understand the *ART* of any particular modality's usage within its own unique context of WHY, HOW, and WHEN. By truly understanding the details of any tool, it is easier to know how to wield and combine multiple ones, fitting them together into a larger picture of optimum health and healing.

A BRIEF REVIEW OF INTEGRATIVE MODALITIES AND ROLES IN POOR PERFORMANCE AND SPORTS MEDICINE
Traditional Chinese (Asian) Medicine

The evidence for the use of acupuncture for sports medicine, performance, and rehabilitation issues is quite extensive in the human field, but is still considered lacking in the veterinary world. Currently, there are 2 approaches toward adding acupuncture. One is using more traditional approaches and techniques (including herbs, food therapy, and fascial manual therapies such as *tui-na* or *gua-sha*) based on the centuries-old, Traditional Asian (Chinese, Tibetan, Nepalese, Korean, Japanese) medical precepts developed or modified for animals. The other is a more modern, evidence-based approach using only acupuncture with needles or laser. It is the experiential opinion of the author that while Medical Acupuncture can be effectively integrated with more conventional treatments for equine sports medicine and rehabilitation problems, adding the more Traditional Asian pattern diagnostics and accompanying treatment options gives the equine clinician more tools to problem-solve vague and challenging performance issues.[7]

One tool that TCVM can provide the practitioner in evaluating poor performance issues is what is a body scan. This is a technique of applying both static and dynamic digital pressure along the various muscles and acupuncture channel anatomic locations to evaluate tone and sensitivity. This sweeping technique with focused palpation can often quickly isolate previously unrecognized areas of muscle hypertonicity, textural changes, scarring, and soreness, helping to identify problems from both a Chinese sports medicine as well as a more conventional biomechanical evaluation.[8]

Chinese herbal formulas specifically are also selected according to the TCVM physiologic pattern.[9,10] Since herbal formulas are prescribed by TCVM clinical sign patterns that include ALL organ systems, herbs may be beneficial for vague performance problems that might fit a particular TCVM physiologic pattern. However, Chinese herbal formulas are complex and competition testing results are mostly unknown. It is recommended that Chinese herba formula use be limited to only those horses not in active competition or only after a substantial withdrawal period before returning to competition.

Food therapy is an integral part of Asian medicine. Various foods have been designated with a particular thermal nature (hot, warm, neutral, cool, cold) over years of clinical usage. Some foods are also considered supportive of various aspects of Chinese physiologic patterning (Blood, Qi, Yin, or Yang supportive). For example, oats are considered warming, and barley is considered cooling, therefore, a veterinary practitioner treating a performance horse may use a feed with more barley in the summer if the horse tends to overheat and more oats in the winter if an older horse is stiffer in the cold. A veterinary practitioner integrating Traditional Asian medicine may also alter feeds in a horse with stamina or fatigue issues to fit the apparent Chinese clinical sign pattern.

For example in adding a more TCVM approach, suppose a veterinary practitioner is presented with chronic tendonitis in a competition horse. The tendon problem has been identified with modern diagnostics and treated with conventional means, even possibly with Medical Acupuncture point selection that has been shown to help with pain, circulation, and healing of the equine distal limb. But what if the tendon is not healing as it should? Trying to promote healing and support collagen regeneration in a horse scheduled for competitions can be frustrating. Adding Traditional Asian (specifically Chinese) medicine by identifying the Traditional Chinese subcategories of dysfunction in that animal can provide the clinician with other options for treatment. Using Traditional Chinese pattern recognition, chronic tendon problems also can be broken down into at least 2 categories.[11]

- Blood Deficiencies: This subcategory is associated with the inability to provide nourishment to the "sinews" or organized connective tissue structures and does not necessarily indicate anemia in the conventional sense. In TCVM, connective tissue problems are related to Liver function physiology (NOTE: to differentiate between conventional medicine and TCVM, organ and dysfunction names are capitalized to denote the TCVM descriptor). The Traditional Chinese veterinary practitioner would recognize this state using traditional techniques for evaluating the tongue color (in this case paler than average) and pulse quality (ie, careful comparative palpation of either carotid or transverse facial arteries would find the left side having a weaker pulse, even possibly with a thinner diameter than the right pulse), as well as a detailed history, physical examination, and evaluation of the horse's behavior. Blood Deficiency animals are often fatigued with low stamina or energy. In TCVM, this would be treated with combinations of acupuncture techniques known to stimulate function (moxa, B-12, laser), herbs focused traditionally toward Blood support, food that is known to support Blood production, and *tui-na* or *gua-sha* protocols that stimulate the fascial pathways from the torso toward the limbs.

- Liver Qi Stagnation: This pattern is related to the inability of the Liver to transport Qi (function)[12] support to the body's connective tissue or sinews. A TCVM practitioner would once again use history, examination, and behavior as well as tongue and pulse evaluations. In this case, the Liver Qi Stagnation horse would be irritable and restless, its tongue that would have a lavender tone on the sides, and arterial pulses would be considered "wiry" or hitting more strongly than average against the fingers. Acupoint selection and method of treatment of this TCVM diagnosis would be different than for the Blood Deficiency. Herbal formulas would contain herbs more specific for liver support (for example, bupleurum), food would focus more on forage with less carbohydrates, and manual therapy protocols would concentrate on passive stretching of limbs and spinal musculature.

Note that in both situations, the ENTIRE animal is evaluated, including behavior and demeanor—treatment protocols are not determined just on the presence of a poorly healing tendon.

Medical Acupuncture/Acupressure

This more modern acupuncture application is primarily used for the treatment of pain, inflammation and to promote healing. As with TCVM, there is a shortage of evidence for the use of particular groupings of acupoints in horses since many acupoint recipes are borrowed from the human medical world.[13–15] However, recent studies have shown that acupuncture improves the metabolism of Thoroughbred race horses,[16] alters equine vagosympathetic tone, decreases cortisol levels during a startle response,[17] and may be a beneficial addition for pain control.[18]

Ayurvedic Medicine

Ayurvedic treatises primarily focus on the restoration of health (or diagnosis of disease) by evaluating the balance between the 3 *doushas* (or constitutions) of *kapha*, *pitta* and *vata*, then prescribing treatment via animal environmental management, food and herbal treatments.[19] There is significant active research occurring both in the human and veterinary fields regarding efficacy and safety of specific herbal components commonly found in Ayurvedic formulas, of which ashwaganda (*Withania somnifera*) and turmeric (*Curcuma longa*) are the most commonly available for equine use.[20,21] Ongoing research includes evaluating various Ayurvedic herbs in the role of bioenhancers that can increase bioavailability and bio-efficacy in various classes of veterinary drugs including antibiotics, antifugals and antivirals, as well as various nutriceuticals.[22] Many Ayurvedic herbs used both in the horse and human have been shown to modulate adaptogenic responses as well as gastric motility.[23] A horse with vague clinical signs related to poor performance could be evaluated and treated using Ayurvedic concepts by a trained practitioner. But, since most Ayurvedic approaches involve the use of herbs, the same caution and warning given for Chinese herbal formulas in competitive horses apply to Ayurvedic herbs as well.

Chiropractic

Chiropractic involves the application of short lever, specifically directed, high velocity thrusts to a joint to restore its motion. Chiropractic is a recognized and common musculoskeletal treatment focusing on restoring mobility to spinal and extraspinal joints. Chiropractic is probably one of the most called on integrative modalities besides acupuncture for treating poor performance and maintenance of musculoskeletal health in the performance animal. Chiropractic has quite a bit of research specifically evaluating efficacy and safety in the horse. Focused evaluation of chiropractic therapy for neck pain,[24] flexibility and performance,[25,26] back pain and motion[27,28] shows some potential improvement in movement and flexibility that helped performance and diminished pain. However, a recent meta-analysis review of equine chiropractic research concluded that due to the variations in study qualities, it was difficult to make hard conclusions regarding chiropractic efficacy despite studies demonstrating that chiropractic beneficially altered spinal mechanical nociceptive thresholds better than massage or phenylbutazone.[29,30] A multimodal approach using both low-level laser therapy in combination with chiropractic improved flexibility, muscle hypertonicity, pain, and trunk stiffness in Quarter Horses better than either modality by itself.[31]

While there are several chiropractic examination techniques, the equine chiropractic examination in general focuses on total body movement integration. In cases of poor performance of unknown origin, this whole-body approach can often discover and treat underlying, low-grade soft tissue pain or musculoskeletal dysfunction, for example, loss of full joint range-of-motion. Applying short-lever, high-velocity chiropractic adjustments near musculoskeletal areas with high-neuronal signaling pathways may trigger nerve reflexes responsible for changing muscle length. This input is thought to play an important role in returning the musculoskeletal system into symmetry by both releasing muscle hypertonicity and allowing muscles under tension to shorten back to ideal length. This may account for the improvements seen in flexibility, stiffness, pain, and decreasing muscle hypertonicity.

Myofascial Therapies

New research regarding fascia and its body-wide interconnectedness must be inserted into the existing musculoskeletal models of muscles, tendons, and ligaments. The human physical therapy world has been exploring the role that kinetic or functional fascial chains (connecting force lines) may play in integrating global body movement.[32-35] Recent research is showing that the same interconnectedness of fascial force lines or "chains" may also exist in animals.[36,37] Further work is certainly needed, but the possibilities that fascial dysfunctions in one area of the body could have effects in more distant locations are intriguing and could revolutionize the ability of the veterinary practitioner to use chiropractic (and other manual therapies) in locating and treating areas of dysfunction or pain contributing to poor performance.

Osteopathy

Osteopathy is based on the health and disease evaluation of a patient considered as a whole unit of body, mind, and spirit capable of self-regulating and self-healing.[38-40] Its use in veterinary medicine is poorly defined with very little research. Chiropractic and osteopathy have similar approaches to whole body health by focusing on the musculoskeletal system; however, Osteopathic techniques often involve blends of tissue mobilization, lymphatic massage, strain/counterstrain movements, and myofascial techniques.[39,40] At this time, research in equine osteopathy is limited in quality, but a couple of studies have shown decreased heart and respiratory rates with osteopathic manipulation.[41] Cortisol levels as well as other blood parameters such as RBC, HGB, HCT, WBC and lymphocyte absolute number are also affected by osteopathic manipulation.[42] A review of manual therapy techniques in the horse concluded that while there is plenty of anecdotal data of positive outcome, there are few, quality controlled studies to allow for definitive conclusions on effectiveness for various equine musculoskeletal conditions as well as treatment parameters such as technique and frequency of application.[43]

Western Herbal Medicine

The use of Western-based herbs in horses is common and often conducted without veterinary input. Clients may try treating their own horse performance issues, such as using Boswellia as a joint antiinflammatory or marshmallow for potential ulcers, long before including a veterinarian in the process. Herbs, however, can provide some assistance with a variety of poor performance issues, including respiratory, gastrointestinal, and musculoskeletal problems.

Herbs can be adulterated with other poor quality and ineffective substances. Additionally, some herbs could be mixed together when horse owners combine different supplements and create interactions or overdosing. The author had a case in an older eventing horse where it was evident from the history of epistaxis and during a blood draw that the horse was having an issue with delayed clotting. Upon the inspection of the supplements, the owner had been combining several "geriatric tonics" that when combined probably had excessive turmeric combined with Jerusalem artichoke and olive leaf. All are herbs that can interfere with clotting. All of the formulas were stopped and the clotting issue gradually went away over several weeks. Veterinarians need to be aware that additional issues may arise as feed companies look at certain herbs as palatants for various horse diets without perhaps understanding what the herbs might do medicinally when not given as stand-alone.[44]

There are many Western herbs that can be safely used over time.[45] Whether any of them have any effect on poor performance issues from respiratory, cardiovascular, endocrine, or musculoskeletal issues is unclear from the literature. Making a link from an underlying deficiency in overall vitality and health (eg, metabolism, immunity), to poor performance is difficult to make from a scientific and measurable perspective, yet, is probably one that veterinary clinicians may face every day. Numerous Western herbs available for horses may have actions at the level of underlying homeostatic functions.[23,46–50] Whether having actions at this level justifies usage without appropriate safety studies remains to be seen. It is possible with future research that more specific usage and safety protocol parameters for various common herbs will be found. For example, recent work using garlic has found that despite the benefits referenced above, some cases of Heinz Body anemia can occur.[51]

Homeopathy

Perhaps one of the most controversial and polarizing integrative medical traditions involves the use of ultra-dilute homeopathic medicine. Homeopathy's greatest primary criticism has revolved around the fact that remedies are so dilute as to have no measurable amount of the original substance remaining. Therefore, homeopathic remedies are often considered antithetical to the current model of drug and receptor, although new biophysics (Quantum, nanoparticles, water organization) research is demonstrating other potential mechanisms of action.[52–56] Additionally, as with many integrative therapies, there is a shortage of quality research, and what is present is confusing and sometimes contradictory, even in the presence of meta-analytical evaluations.[57,58]

Commercial remedies are available as diluted, water–alcohol tinctures, or the tincture may be sprayed onto lactose or sucrose pellets, allowed to dry then sold as various sizes of pellets. The preferential method of administration with animals is directly onto the gum or tongue. Higher potency remedies (more dilute) are treated as if they have a stronger physiologic effect (due to increased succussions or mixing affecting water structure). Homeopathic remedies are considered safe with minimal side-effects. Since a complete body clinical sign picture is used to select a homeopathic remedy, remedies are selected to treat an animal with greater individualization, even in cases of vague performance issues. When selecting remedies, not only can separate, specific clinical signs from multiple body systems be included in creating any one individual's pattern (eg, sensitive tendon, swollen muscle, right side vs left side, wet or dry cough, or tendency to colic with stress), but consideration is also given to how any particular clinical sign is affected by other factors including weather and exercise (eg, better or worse in one type of weather temperature over another, better or worse with changes in barometric pressure, or better or worse with exercise).

PRACTICAL DECISION-MAKING USING INTEGRATIVE THERAPIES

The choices of any practitioner in deciding what integrative modalities to use will be dependent on that particular practitioner's knowledge, training, treatment biases, and availability to veterinary colleagues trained in specific techniques. The application of integrative modalities to any one case will vary and be more tailored to individual needs and client preferences. Whether or not a case of vague performance problems is treated only with external therapies such as acupuncture or chiropractic versus internal ones such as Chinese, Western herbs may depend on availability, cost, knowledge-base, and in the competitive horse, possible conflict with drug testing.

Presented with a case of mild to moderate exercise intolerance (often perceived by a client as stiffness, labored movement or fatiguing sooner than expected), especially in a horse that seems to be moving adequately, once a history and physical examination have ruled out the obvious such as nutritional deficiencies, myopathies or cardiopulmonary issues, a practitioner can simply start by evaluating the horse using chiropractic or osteopathic techniques to evaluate for body soreness and functional straightness. The clinician can start with either chiropractic or osteopathic treatment to see what kind of response occurs. Often increased stiffness or pain from asymmetric movement can lead to increased movement effort and decreased stamina. Acupuncture can also be considered a primary treatment used alone or in conjunction with a structural modality. Most integrative veterinary practitioners will tailor the frequency of treatment to the health and competitive needs of the individual. Regular treatments might be initially needed until an individual has healed from injury or reached a different level of conditioning that allows for maintenance. Horses that have transitioned from crisis management to maintenance may have treatments timed to be most effective for competitions or travel. Horses that show definite seasonal worsening (such as when temperatures grow cooler), especially geriatric ones where osteoarthritis could be contributing to poor performance, may benefit from warming acupuncture with a laser or moxa, addition of warming herbs such as ginger, and switching feed from barley to oats in advance of seasonal changes.

In the geriatric horse with osteoarthritis or one with post injury or illness problems, secondary treatments after the use of acupuncture and chiropractic or osteopathy can include more sustained use of daily-fed Western, Chinese or Ayurvedic herbs. Homeopathic remedies can be added in an as needed basis depending on how well the specific tissue is healing and what the horse is doing in terms of progress and exercise. Homeopathic remedies may need to be changed as healing progresses. *Arnica* may be an appropriate remedy early on in a serious muscle injury, but *silicea* may need to be given if the injury starts to develop significant scar tissue.

SUMMARY

The use of integrative therapies is growing more commonplace and widespread in equine veterinary medicine, especially in cases of poor performance and sports medicine. Adding one or more modalities such as Traditional Asian Medicine (acupuncture, food therapy, traditional herbal formulas, manual therapy), Medical acupuncture, Ayurvedic medicine, chiropractic, osteopathy, western herbs, and homeopathy, can provide practitioners with additional means to help with the diagnosis and treatment of vague cases of poor performance. The treatment possibilities available to the clinician when adding integrative therapies with conventional approaches are many and create more tools for changing challenging and frustrating cases into scenarios with more positive outcomes for all involved.

DISCLOSURE

The author has no conflicts to disclose.

REFERENCES

1. Keller P, Vanwesenbeeck I, Hudders L, et al. Horse owners' attitudes towards and motivators for using complementary and alternative veterinary medicine. Vet Rec 2021;189(2):e303.
2. Wilson JM, McKenzie E, Duesterdieck-Zellmer K. International Survey Regarding the Use of Rehabilitation Modalities in Horses. Front Vet Sci 2018;5:120.
3. Loving NS. Survey of horse owners regarding complementary therapies. Equimanagement. 2018. Available at: https://equimanagement.com/articles/survey-of-horse-owners-regarding-complementary-therapies/. Accessed June 13, 22.
4. Thirkell J, Hyland R. A survey examining attitude towards equine complementary therapies for the treatment of musculoskeletal injuries. J Eq Vet Sci 2017;59:82–7.
5. Meredith K, Bolwell CV, Rogers CW, et al. The use of allied health therapies on competition horses in the North Island of New Zealand. NZ Vet J 2011;59:123–7.
6. Hinchcliff KW, Geor RJ. Integrative physiology of exercise. In: Hinchcliff KW, Kaneps A, Geor RJ, editors. Equine sports medicine & surgery. Edinburgh: Elsevier; 2004. p. 3–8.
7. Le Jeune S, Henneman K, May K. Acupuncture and Equine Rehabilitation. Vet Clin North Am Equine Pract 2016;32(1):73–85.
8. Le Jeune SS, Jones JH. Prospective study on the correlation of positive acupuncture scans and lameness in 102 performance horses. Am J Trad Chin Vet Med 2014;9(2):33–41.
9. Chen JK, Chen TT. Chinese medical herbology and pharmacology. CA: Art of Medicine Press; 2004.
10. Chen JK, Chen TT, Beebe S, et al. Chinese herbal formulas for veterinarians. CA: Art of Medicine Press; 2012.

11. Callison M. Acupuncture Sports Medicine. Acusport Education 2019.

12. Kendall DE. Dao of Chinese medicine: understanding an ancient healing art. Oxford, UK: Oxford University Press; 2002.

13. Ma YT. Biomedical acupuncture for sports & trauma rehabilitation: dry needling techniques. ???: Churchill Livingstone Elsevier; 2011.

14. Ma YT, Ma M, Cho ZH. Biomedical acupuncture for pain management: an integrative approach. Edinburgh: Churchill Livingstone Elsevier; 2005.

15. Reaves W, Bong C. The acupuncture handbook of sports injuries & pain: a four-step approach to treatment. Boulder, CO: Hidden Needle Press; 2009.

16. Angeli AL, Luna SPL. Aquapuncture improves metabolic capacity in Thoroughbred horses. J Eq Vet Sci 2008;28(9):525–31.

17. Villas-Boas JD, Dias DPM, Trigo PI, et al. Acupuncture affects autonomic and endocrine but not behavioural responses induced by startle in horses. Evid-Based Comp Alt Med; 2015. p. 219579. https://doi.org/10.1155/2015/219579. Accessed May 30, 2022.

18. Mama KR, Hector RC. Therapeutic developments in equine pain management. Vet J 2019;247:50–6.

19. Mazars G. Traditional veterinary medicine in India. Rev Sci Tech 1994;13(2):433–51.

20. Priyanka G, Anil Kumar B, Lakshman M, et al. Adaptogenic and Immunomodulatory Activity of Ashwagandha Root Extract: An Experimental Study in an Equine Model. Front Vet Sci 2020;7:541112.

21. EFSA Panel on Additives and Products or Substances used in Animal Feed (FEE-DAP), Bampidis V, Azimonti G, et al. Safety and efficacy of turmeric extract, turmeric oil, turmeric oleoresin and turmeric tincture from *Curcuma longa* L. rhizome when used as sensory additives in feed for all animal species. EFSA J 2020;18(6):e06146.

22. Yurdakok-Dikmen B, Turgut Y, Filazi A. Herbal Bioenhancers in Veterinary Phytomedicine. Front Vet Sci 2018;5:249.

23. Rege NN, Thatte UM, Dahanukar SA. Adaptogenic properties of six rasayana herbs used in Ayurvedic medicine. Phytother Res 1999;13(4):275–91.

24. Story MR, Haussler KK, Nout-Lomas YS, et al. Equine Cervical Pain and Dysfunction: Pathology, Diagnosis and Treatment. Animals (Basel) 2021;11(2):422.

25. Haussler KK. Joint Mobilization and Manipulation for the Equine Athlete. Vet Clin North Am Equine Pract 2016;32(1):87–101.

26. Haussler KK. Equine Manual Therapies in Sport Horse Practice. Vet Clin North Am Equine Pract 2018;34(2):375–89.

27. Gomez Alvarez CB, L'ami JJ, Moffat D, et al. Effect of chiropractic manipulations on the kinematics of back and limbs in horses with clinically diagnosed back problems. Equine Vet J 2008;40(2):153–9.

28. Haussler KK, Erb HN. Pressure algometry: Objective assessment of back pain and effects of chiropractic treatment. Proc Am Assoc Equine Pract 2003;49:66–70. New Orleans, LA, USA. 21–25.

29. Haussler KK, Hesbach AL, Romano L, et al. A Systematic Review of Musculoskeletal Mobilization and Manipulation Techniques Used in Veterinary Medicine. Animals (Basel) 2021;11(10):2787.

30. Sullivan KA, Hill AE, Haussler KK. The effects of chiropractic, massage and phenylbutazone on spinal mechanical nociceptive thresholds in horses without clinical signs. Equine Vet J 2008;40(1):14–20.

31. Haussler KK, Manchon PT, Donnell JR, et al. Effects of Low-Level Laser Therapy and Chiropractic Care on Back Pain in Quarter Horses. J Equine Vet Sci 2020;86: 102891.

32. Krause F, Wilke J, Vogt L, et al. Intermuscular force transmission along myofascial chains: a systematic review. J Anat 2016;228(6):910–8.

33. Schliep R. Fascia as a body-wide tensional network: anatomy, biomechanics and physiology. In: Schliep R, Baker A, editors. Fascia in sport & movement. Edinburgh: Handspring Publishing; 2015. p. 3–11.

34. Myers TW. Anatomy Trains: myofascial meridians for manual therapists & movement professionals. 4th edn. Elsevier; 2014.

35. Wilke J, Niederer D, Vogt L, et al. Remote effects of lower limb stretching: preliminary evidence for myofascial connectivity? J Sports Sci 2016;34(22):2145–8.

36. Schultz RM, Due T. Elbrøond Equine myofascial kinetic lines – for professionals. Kalmar, Sweden: Leanders Grafiska AB; 2021.

37. Ahmed W, Kulikowska M, Ahlmann T, et al. A comparative multi-site and whole-body assessment of fascia in the horse and dog: a detailed histological investigation. J Anat 2019;235(6):1065–77.

38. Eaton JA, Bates BP, Willard FH. Osteopathic medicine. Orthop Nurs 1991;10(1): 51–61.

39. Seffinger MA, Hruby RJ, Rogers FJ, et al. Philosophy of Osteopathic Medicine in Seffinger MA. In: Hruby RJ, Willard FH, Licciardone J, editors. Foundations for osteopathic medicine. 4th edn. Philadelphia: Wolters Kluwer Health/Lippincott Williams & Wilkins; 2018. p. 2–18.

40. Gunnar Brolinson P, McGinley SM, Kerger S. Osteopathic manipulative medicine and the athlete. Curr Sports Med Rep 2008;7(1):49–56.

41. Babarskaitė G, Vokietytė-Vilėniškė G. Osteopathic manual therapy in equine. In: Gabrielė J, editor. IHS [international health Sciences] Conference: abstract book [29-30 April] 2021/Students' scientific Society of Lithuanian University of health Sciences. Kaunas: Lithuanian University of Health Sciences; 2021.

42. Vokietytė-Vilėniškė G, Žilaitis V, Miknienė Z. Changes of cortisol and whole blood level induced by equine osteopathic treatment. International [8th] conference of young scientists" Young scientists for advance of agriculture": abstracts:[14 November 2019, Vilnius, Lithuania]. Vilnius: Lithuanian Academy of Sciences; 2019.

43. Haussler KK. Review of manual therapy techniques in equine practice. J Equine Vet Sci 2009;29(12):849–69.

44. Stachurska A, Tkaczyk E, Różańska-Boczula M, et al. Horses' Response to a Novel Diet: Different Herbs Added to Dry, Wet or Wet-Sweetened Oats. Animals (Basel) 2022;12(11):1334.

45. Williams CA, Lamprecht ED. Some commonly fed herbs and other functional foods in equine nutrition: a review. Vet J 2008;178(1):21–31.

46. Saastamoinen M, Särkijärvi S, Hyyppä S. Garlic (*Allium Sativum*) Supplementation Improves Respiratory Health but Has Increased Risk of Lower Hematologic Values in Horses. Animals (Basel) 2019;9(1):13.

47. Suagee-Bedore JK, Shen Y, Porr S, et al. Impacts of DigestaWell NRG Supplementation on Post Exercise Muscle Soreness in Unconditioned Horses, a Pilot Study. J Equine Vet Sci 2021;101:103455.

48. Mbarki S, Alimi H, Bouzenna H, et al. Phytochemical study and protective effect of Trigonella foenum graecum (Fenugreek seeds) against carbon tetrachloride-induced toxicity in liver and kidney of male rat. Biomed Pharmacother 2017;88: 19–26.

49. Nagamma T, Konuri A, Bhat KM, et al. Prophylactic effect of *Trigonella foenum-graecum L.* seed extract on inflammatory markers and histopathological changes in high-fat-fed ovariectomized rats. J Tradit Complement Med 2021;12(2):131–40.

50. Axmann S, Hummel K, Nöbauer K, et al. Pharmacokinetics of harpagoside in horses after intragastric administration of a Devil's claw (Harpagophytum procumbens) extract. J Vet Pharmacol Ther 2019;42(1):37–44.

51. Pearson W, Boermans HJ, Bettger WJ, et al. Association of maximum voluntary dietary intake of freeze-dried garlic with Heinz body anemia in horses. Am J Vet Res 2005;66(3):457–65.

52. Ullman D. Exploring Possible Mechanisms of Hormesis and Homeopathy in the Light of Nanopharmacology and Ultra-High Dilutions. Dose Response 2021;19(2). 15593258211022983.

53. Hwang SG, Hong JK, Sharma A, et al. Exclusion zone and heterogeneous water structure at ambient temperature. PLoS One 2018;13(4):e0195057.

54. Bellavite P, Marzotto M, Olioso D, et al. High-dilution effects revisited. 1. Physico-chemical aspects. Homeopathy 2014;103(1):4–21.

55. Bellavite P, Marzotto M, Olioso D, et al. High-dilution effects revisited. 2. Pharmacodynamic mechanisms. Homeopathy 2014;103(1):22–43.

56. Montagnier L, Aïssa J, Ferris S, et al. Electromagnetic signals are produced by aqueous nanostructures derived from bacterial DNA sequences. Interdiscip Sci 2009;1(2):81–90.

57. Mathie RT. Controlled clinical studies of homeopathy. Homeopathy 2015;104(4):328–32.

58. Hahn RG. Homeopathy: meta-analyses of pooled clinical data. Forsch Komplementmed 2013;20(5):376–81.

Preventative Care
Managing the Geriatric Horse with Integrative Therapies

Edward Boldt Jr, DVM

KEYWORDS

- Geriatric • Equine • Integrative therapies • Acupuncture • Chiropractic

KEY POINTS

- Horses 15 years of age and older now account for a significant portion of the equine population.
- Maintaining these aging horses is a challenge, especially because of the chronicity of some healthy issues.
- Integrative therapies are beneficial to provide diagnostic and therapeutic options for the preventative care and health maintenance of these patients.

INTRODUCTION

Not long ago horses living into their 20s was considered a long life. Now it is routine to see horses live into their 30s and beyond. The Equine 2015 study by the US Department of Agriculture found that 11% of the equid population was 20 years old or older.[1] A study done in the United Kingdom showed horses 15 years old and older accounted for 29% of the population, whereas a study done at University of Kentucky, Gluck Equine Research Center showed horses 15 years and older account for a significant portion of the equine population in the United States.[2,3]

This increase in longevity of the equine population is caused by advances in management of these senior horses. Maintaining these geriatric horses is a challenge, especially because of the chronicity of some issues. Integrative therapies are beneficial in helping the equine veterinarian address some of these chronic issues. This article shows the potential use of integrative therapies as part of the overall management of the geriatric horse.

Performance Horse Complementary Medicine Services, PLLC, 6520 E County Road 44, Fort Collins, CO 80524, USA
E-mail address: Dr.Ed@horsvet.com

Vet Clin Equine 38 (2022) 475–483
https://doi.org/10.1016/j.cveq.2022.06.005
0749-0739/22/© 2022 Elsevier Inc. All rights reserved.
vetequine.theclinics.com

USE OF INTEGRATIVE THERAPIES AS A DIAGNOSTIC AID

The geriatric patient should undergo a conventional physical examination as with any equine patient. Any issues noted requiring further diagnostics (eg, blood work, radiographs) should be performed. However, integrative therapies, such as acupuncture and spinal manipulation (chiropractic), are useful diagnostic aids.

Certain combinations of reactive acupuncture points identified on cutaneous stimulation or palpation (eg, flinching, muscle twitch, withdrawal responses) can suggest areas of the body to examine more closely. The identification and localization of reactive acupuncture points does not constitute a specific diagnosis or indicate local tissue pathology, but suggests that these regions may warrant further examination. Different combinations of reactive points are evaluated to suggest a potential acupuncture issue within a body region or tissue. Some examples include:

1. Hoof: reactivity at LI-18, ST-10, LU-1, and PC-1[a] suggests a hoof issue.
2. Carpus: reactivity at LI-16 to LI-17 suggests a carpal issue.
   a. If the carpal articulations have no signs of inflammation, response to palpation, and passive joint motion, then the digital flexor tendons and proximal suspensory ligament are palpated and examined in more detail.
3. Hock: reactivity at BL-39, BL-40, GB-DTC, and the so-called Churchill point (located at the caudal aspect of the base of the medial splint and medial aspect carpometacarpal joint) suggests hock involvement.
4. Stifle: reactivity in the area from BL-36 to BL-38, along with KI-10 and GB-28 suggests stifle problems.
   a. Detailed palpation of the stifle usually confirms joint effusion or pain.

The addition of acupuncture point and channel palpation into a conventional physical examination may provide another means to better identify horses with subtle musculoskeletal or performance issues.[4] Although the examination of acupuncture points is used as a quick method of identifying tissues or body regions that should undergo further detailed examination and diagnostic tests (eg, flexion tests, radiographs), as indicated, the acupuncture evaluation is not a substitute for a full conventional lameness examination.[5]

The inclusion of joint motion palpation or other chiropractic techniques is useful in locating areas of decreased range of motion, pain, and muscle hypertonicity. These areas can then also be further examined from a conventional standpoint and any other diagnostics (eg, ultrasound, radiographs) performed.

FIVE CLINICALLY RELEVANT ISSUES IN THE GERIATRIC HORSE
Navicular Disease

Signs of navicular disease (podotrochlosis, palmar heel pain) can often be identified in geriatric horses. Affected horses are often retired competition horses that have been dealing with chronic foot pain for years. Most horses have undergone conventional diagnostics that include lameness examination, diagnostic nerve blocks, radiographs, and in some cases MRI. Many affected horses have been treated with corrective shoeing and nonsteroidal anti-inflammatory drugs (NSAIDs), often along with corticosteroid injections of the navicular bursa or coffin joint.

Acupuncture and Chinese herbal therapy is beneficial in these patients as an adjunctive therapy. The author uses a five-needle technique within the affected front

---

[a] All International Veterinary Acupuncture Society equine point locations are found in **Table 1**.

Table 1 Equine acupuncture points (from the International Veterinary Acupuncture Society)	
LU-1	In the deep depression in the center of the muscle belly of the pectoralis descendens, at the level of the 1st intercostal space.
LU-7	In the depression on the medial surface of the radius, 1.5 cun proximal to the most medial prominence of the styloid process. This point is 0.5 cun distal to the level of PC-6.
LU-11	In the depression on the palmaromedial aspect of the front foot, just proximal to the coronary band, approximately two-thirds of the distance from the dorsal midline of the coronary band to the palmar border of the medial bulb of the heel.
LI-1	In the depression on the dorsomedial aspect of the front foot, just proximal to the coronary band, approximately one-third of the distance from the dorsal midline of the coronary band to the palmar border of the medial bulb of the heel.
LI-18	In the depression on the cranioventral border of the cleidomastoideus portion of the brachiocephalicus m., in an area cranioventral to the junction of the 2nd and 3rd cervical vertebrae, dorsal to the jugular vein. Some authors use the junction of a line that runs parallel to the ventral aspect of the mandible, and its intersection with the cervical vertebral column (with the head extended).
ST-10	In the depression in the muscular groove between the sternocephalicus and the cleidomastoideus branch of the brachiocephalicus mm., cranioventral to the junction of the 5th and 6th cervical vertebrae.
ST-35	In the large depression ventral to the ventral border of the patella and between the middle and lateral patellar ligaments. ST-35 and medial XIYAN together make up the traditional point, XIYAN (Knee Eyes).
ST-36	In the depression just lateral to the tibial crest, in the muscular groove between the tibialis cranialis and long digital extensor mm., 2 cun distal to the proximal edge of the tibial crest. An alternate location is as in the canine, which puts it in the middle of the muscle belly of the tibialis cranialis, but because of the lack of acceptance by the horse, the previously mentioned location is used. The direction of needle insertion for this point is craniolateral to caudomedial, whereas that for the alternate point is cranial to caudal; thus both insertions arrive at the same point.
SP-9	In the depression just ventral to the medial condyle of the tibia, caudal to the caudal border of the tibia, over the popliteus m. and cranial to the saphenous vein.
HT-7	In the depression on the medial surface of the radius, just cranial to the cranial border of the flexor carpi ulnaris m., at the level of the dorsal aspect of the accessory carpal bone (superficial location), with the deeper location between the flexor carpi ulnaris and superficial digital flexor mm. Needle insertion is at a 90° angle to the skin surface.
HT-9	In the depression on the palmarolateral aspect of the front foot, just proximal to the coronary band, approximately two-thirds of the distance from the dorsal midline of the coronary band to the palmar border of the lateral bulb of the heel.
SI-1	In the depression on the dorsolateral aspect of the front foot, just proximal to the coronary band, approximately one-third of the distance from the dorsal midline of the coronary band to the palmar border of the lateral bulb of the heel.
SI-9	In the large depression along the caudal border of the deltoid m. and between the long and lateral heads of the triceps brachii m.

(continued on next page)

Table 1 (continued)	
BL-11	In the depression just cranial to the craniodorsal border of the scapular cartilage, 1.5 cun lateral to the dorsal midline, over the cervical portion of the trapezius m.
BL-18	In the depression 3 cun lateral to the dorsal midline, this point has 2 locations: in the 13th and 14th intercostal spaces, in the muscular groove between the longissimus thoracis and iliocostalis thoracis mm.
BL-21	In the depression 3 cun lateral to the dorsal midline, in the depression caudal to the 18th (last) rib, between the 18th thoracic and 1st lumbar vertebrae (thoracolumbar junction), in the muscular groove between the longissimus lumborum and iliocostalis lumborum mm.
BL-26	In the depression 3 cun lateral to the dorsal midline, between the spinous processes of the 6th lumbar (or L5, if L6 is missing) and the 1st sacral vertebrae.
BL-36	In the depression in the muscular groove between the biceps femoris and semitendinosus mm., 2 cun distal to the tuber ischii (ischial tuber).
BL-37	In the depression in the muscular groove between the biceps femoris and the semitendinosus mm., 5 cun distal to the tuber ischii (ischial tuber). This is 3 cun distal to BL-36.
BL-38	In the depression in the muscular groove between the biceps femoris and semitendinosus mm., 8 cun distal to the tuber ischii (ischial tuber). This is 3 cun distal to BL-37.
BL-39	In the depression just medial to the caudal border of the caudal division of the biceps femoris m., at the ventral end of the muscular groove between the biceps femoris and semitendinosus mm. This point is found just lateral to BL-40 with the stifle flexed.
BL-40	In the depression at the midpoint of the transverse crease of the popliteal fossa, in the caudal division of the biceps femoris and the semitendinosus mm. This point is found more easily with the stifle flexed.
BL-60	In the depression on the lateral aspect of the hock area, in the middle of the webbed area cranial to the calcaneal tendon, at the level of the tip of the tuber calcanei (calcanean tuber).
KI-3	In the depression on the medial aspect of the hock area, in the middle of the webbed area cranial to the calcaneal tendon, at the level of the tip of the tuber calcanei (calcanean tuber). This point is medial and slightly distal to BL-60.
KI-10	In the depression between the semitendinosus and gracilis mm., at the level of the popliteal fossa.
PC-1	In the depression on the lateral thorax, caudal to the tip of the olecranon, at the 5th intercostal space, over the ascending pectoral m.
PC-9	In the depression on the palmar midline of the front foot between the bulbs of the heel.
TH-1	In the depression on the dorsal midline of the front foot just proximal to the coronary band.
TH-5	In the depression in the groove between the tendons of the lateral digital extensor and common digital extensor mm., at the level of the midportion of the cranial border of the chestnut. Some authors have placed this point in the depression 2 cun dorsal to the dorsal edge of the ulnar carpal bone.
GB-DTC[a]	In the depression just medial to the most dorsal aspect of the tuber coxae (coxal tuber), on a line drawn at a 90° angle to the dorsal midline and extending to the most dorsal aspect of the tuber coxae.

(continued on next page)

Table 1 (continued)	
GB-27	In the depression just cranial to the midportion of the cranial border of the tuber coxae.
GB-28	In the depression just ventral to the ventral border of the tuber coxae.
GB-39	In the depression 3 cun proximal to the most lateral prominence of the lateral malleolus of the tibia, caudal to the tibial border, cranial to the deep digital flexor m.
LIV-4	In the depression of the dorsal branch of the medial saphenous vein, dorsomedial to the medial branch of the tibialis cranialis m. (cunean tendon), at the level of the distal intertarsal joint.
LIV-8	In the depression caudal to the medial condyle of the femur, cranial to the insertion of the semitendinosus and semimembranosus mm. and caudal to the medial saphenous vein.
Bai Hui[a]	The depression on the dorsal midline in the lumbosacral space.
GV-4	In the depression on the dorsal midline between the spinous processes of the 2nd and 3rd lumbar vertebrae.
Qian Ti Men[a]	In the depression on the front foot, just proximal to the coronary band of the heel bulb, on the inside of the collateral cartilage (relative to the midsagittal plane of the foot). This point has 2 locations per foot, 1 on each heel bulb.

Abbreviations: BL, bladder; DTC, dorsal tuber coxae; GB, gallbladder; GV, governing vessel; HT, heart; KI, kidney; LI, large intestine; LIV, liver; LU, lung; PC, pericardium; SI, small intestine; SP, spleen; ST, stomach; TH, triple heater.

[a] Designated as "Traditional Chinese Veterinary Medicine" points. All other points are based on human transpositional points.

Adapted from The International Veterinary Acupuncture Society, Equine Required Point List with Permission. www.IVAS.org.

feet that uses short acupuncture needles placed at acupoints PC-9, Qian Ti Men, and bilateral points located at the palmar aspect of the medial and lateral heel bulbs along the coronary band (**Fig. 1**) with two additional needles placed in TH-5 on the lateral aspect of the leg at the level of the chestnut in both front limbs (**Fig. 2**). The needles are left in place for 20 minutes. The treatment is repeated every 3 to 7 days for total of three treatments. The horse is then treated twice more at 2-week intervals. Subsequent treatments are dependent on the horse's response but may be monthly or extended out for several months.

In addition to acupuncture, Chinese herbal formulas are also of benefit for horses with signs of navicular disease. The author often adds the formula Hot Hoof I[b] to the treatment regimen. The concentrated formula is added to the feed as a top dressing and fed twice per day for up to 3 months. After 3 months, horses are given 1 month off the formula before starting another 3-month period if needed.

Extracorporeal shock wave therapy can also be used in the more refractory cases of navicular disease. Treatment is applied over the frog per the manufacturer's recommendations using focused shockwave, typically 400 shocks per session every 2 weeks for three sessions.

---

[b] Dr Xie's Jing Tang Herbal Inc, Reddick, FL www.tcvmherbal.com.

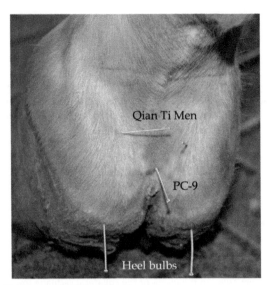

Fig. 1. PC-9, Qian Ti Men, and bilateral heel points.

Chronic Laminitis

Chronic laminitis is a common clinical condition seen in geriatric equines and is caused by a variety of causes. Most affected horses have undergone corrective shoeing or hoof trimming and treatment with various NSAIDs, which has helped to provide some level of comfort or management of the disease process. However, proper shoeing and trimming must be continually reassessed and the overall health of the horse closely monitored. Despite the best efforts to maintain affected horses, geriatric patients can often be susceptible to acute or recurrent laminitic events.

For the stabilize laminitic conditions in affected horse, the author usually prescribes the Chinese herbal formula Hot Hoof I[b]. This is a milder herbal formulation that is used for chronic laminitis once the acute inflammation has been treated and has subsided.[6] The concentrated formula is fed as a top dressing on the feed twice per day. Horses may be maintained on the formula for up to 3 months. Subsequent use is evaluated at that time. Acupuncture can also be applied at acupoint BL-60 for additional pain management (**Fig. 3**).

If an acute laminitic episode does occur, then in addition to conventional treatments typically used, acupuncture points located just above the coronary band (ie, Ting points) in both front feet are stimulated by stabbing the skin with a lancet or hypodermic needle to produce local bleeding (hemoacupuncture) at LU-11, LI-1, TH-1, PC-9, SI-1, and HT-9. Acupoints BL-60 can also be needled bilaterally for additional pain relief. The author also changes the Chinese herbal formula from Hot Hoof I to Hot Hoof II[b] because this formula has more anti-inflammatory effects and is indicated for cases of acute laminitis.[6]

Pituitary Pars Intermedia Dysfunction

Pituitary pars intermedia dysfunction (PPID; equine Cushing disease) is the most common endocrine disease affecting geriatric equines[7] with most horses diagnosed around 20 years of age.[8] Diagnosis typically involves several approaches. In advanced PPID, hypertrichosis (hirsutism) can serve as a diagnosis and has a reported high

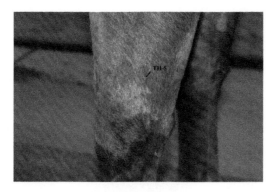

Fig. 2. TH-5.

specificity.[7] Horses with suspected PPID may also be diagnosed with either testing corticotropin levels or by doing a thyrotropin-releasing hormone stimulation test.

Once a horse is diagnosed with PPID, conventional treatment options are often limited. The primary treatment option is pergolide mesylate, which is a dopamine receptor agonist used to restore dopaminergic inhibition of melanotrophs and is the only Food and Drug Administration–approved medication for treating PPID in horses. Some affected horses may also need to be on cyproheptadine, which decreases plasma corticotropin levels and antagonizes serotonin.[7] Horses with advanced PPID and hypertrichosis may require regular body clipping. Alternative treatment options may need to be considered because of owner concerns of high costs for medications and management restrictions, such as the inability to administer medications as prescribed.[9]

Integrative therapies offer additional options to improve the life of the PPID-affected horse and possibly reduce the required dosages of prescribed medications. Traditional Chinese veterinary medicine looks at PPID from the standpoint of three different patterns (Yin deficiency, Qi-Yin deficiency, and Yang deficiency), with the geriatric horse falling primarily into the Yang deficiency pattern. Acupuncture treatment involves needling acupoints BL-26, BL-18, BL-21, ST-36, GV-3, GV-4, CV-4[c], and CV-6[c]. The Chinese herbal formula Rehmannia 14[b] is also added to the treatment as a feed top dressing for up to 3 months.[10]

Osteoarthritis

Osteoarthritis of the carpus, hock, and stifle is a significant cause of lameness in the geriatric horse, which can significantly decrease the quality of life in affected horses. Conventional therapy may include oral administration of NSAIDs and periodic intra-articular corticosteroid injections; however, prolonged use may be associated with significant adverse effects in older horses.

Carpal pain may be addressed by using passive joint range of motion and manipulation to maintain carpal range of motion. Acupuncture points LI-1, SI-9, TH-5, HT-7, LU-7, and BL-11 are stimulated to also help with pain management.

Hock osteoarthritis is treated by stimulating acupoints Bai Hui, BL-60, GB-39, KI-3, and LIV-4. If the tarsal joints have been recently injected with corticosteroids, then it may be beneficial to add extracorporeal shock wave therapy using manufacturer's recommended settings.

---

[c] Xie's Veterinary Acupuncture, Blackwell Publishing, 2007, pp 82–83.

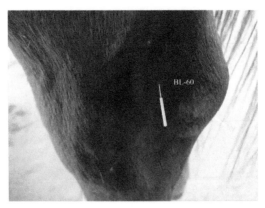

Fig. 3. Acupoint BL-60.

Acupuncture for stifle pain may consist of needling acupoints Bai Hui, ST-35, ST-36, LIV-8, and SP-9. Low-level laser therapy may also be considered as an additional treatment for managing stifle osteoarthritis using the manufacturer's recommended settings.

All of the previously mentioned osteoarthritic conditions may benefit from the use of the Chinese herbal formulas Body Sore and Sang Zhi San.[b]

Axial Skeleton Pain and Stiffness

Many geriatric horses have decreased joint range of motion and pain throughout their neck and back regions. Conventional treatment often consists of the administration of NSAIDs, muscle relaxants (eg, methocarbamol), intra-articular or periarticular injections of corticosteroids, or regional injections using mesotherapy.

In horses with neck and back pain, integrative therapies are of great benefit. The use of joint motion palpation can help to localize areas of decreased range of motion and passive joint mobilization procedures can reduce pain, stiffness, and muscle hypertonicity in affected vertebral regions. Depending on the location of pain, local acupoints that are located primarily along the bladder channel can be dry needled or injected with small volumes (eg, 1–2 mL) of vitamin B_{12} (1000 μg/mL, aquapuncture) into reactive points. Electroacupuncture has also been shown to be beneficial for treating chronic thoracolumbar pain.[11]

PREVENTATIVE CARE USING INTEGRATIVE THERAPY

Along with the routine conventional physical examination, vaccinations, and dental examinations and treatment, geriatric horses can benefit from periodic evaluation and treatments using integrative therapies, such as chiropractic, acupuncture, and active or passive stretching exercises. Joint motion palpation may be used to help localize potential areas of discomfort that may be addressed with joint mobilization or manipulation techniques. Assessing passive and active joint motion may also show that certain stretching exercises are indicated to help maintain joint range of motion, especially through the neck and back regions.

Routine examination of acupoints and channels can help to identify potential disease processes or areas of discomfort that may be alleviated with acupuncture techniques. Horses with chronic, recurrent, or poorly managed conditions (eg, podotrochlosis) can benefit from routine acupuncture treatment. Integrative therapies should be considered as part of the overall health and maintenance plans for geriatric horses.

CLINICS CARE POINTS

- Geriatric patients may benefit from the use of integrative therapies as part of their overall health management.

- Integrative therapies such as acupuncture and chiropractic examinations may aid in localizing areas of the body that may require futher conventional diagnostics.

- Other forms of acupuncture, such as aquapuncture and electroacupuncture, along with the use of Chinese herbal formulas, may also be considered in the treatment of the geriatric horse.

DISCLOSURE

The author has nothing to disclose.

REFERENCES

1. USDA-APHIS-VS-NAHMS. Equine 2015-Baseline Reference of Equine Health and Management in the United States, 2015. 2016.
2. Ireland JL, Clegg PD, McKane SA, et al. A cross-sectional study of geriatric horses in the United Kingdom. Part 1: demographics and management practices. Equine Vet J 2011;43(1):30–6.
3. Herbst A. UK Gluck Equine Research Center launches national survey on horses 15 years and older. 2020. Available at: https://news.ca.uky.edu/article/uk-gluck-equine-research-center-launches-national-survey-horses-aged-15-years-and-older.
4. Alfaro A. Correlation of acupuncture point sensitivity and lesion location in 259 horses. AJTCVM 2014;9(1):83–7.
5. le Jeune S, Jones JH. Prospective study on the correlation of positive acupuncture scans and lameness in 102 performance horses. AJTCVM 2014;9(2):33–41.
6. Xie H, Deng X, Das M. Chinese veterinary herbal handbook. Reddick (FL): Chi Institute of Chinese Medicine; 2000. p. p7–8.
7. Frank N. Pituitary pars intermedia dysfunction. In: Spayberry K, Robinson NE, editors. Robinson's current therapy in equine medicine. 7th edition. St Louis: Elsevier Saunders; 2015. p. 574–7.
8. Wallis C, Harman J. TCVM for equine endocrine and metabolic diseases. In: Xie H, Wedemeyer L, Chrisman C, et al, editors. Practical guide to traditional Chinese veterinary medicine: equine practice. Reddick: Chi Institute Press; 2015. p. 335–59.
9. Carmalt J, Waldner C, Allen A. Equine pituitary pars intermedia dysfunction: an international survey of veterinarians' approach to diagnosis, management, and estimated prevalence. Can J Vet Res 2017;81(4):261–9.
10. Xie H. Acupuncture for internal medicine. In: Xie H, Preast V, editors. Xie's veterinary acupuncture. Ames: Blackwell; 2007. p. 267–308.
11. Xie H, Colahan P, Ott E. Evaluation of electroacupuncture treatment of horses with signs of chronic thoracolumbar pain. JAVMA 2005;227(2):281–6.

Integrative Approach to Neck Pain and Dysfunction

Melinda R. Story, DVM, PhD

KEYWORDS

- Equine • Cervical • Pain • Myofascial examination

KEY POINTS

- Horses experiencing cervical pain and dysfunction may present in a number of different ways and can be difficult to manage.
- A very thorough physical assessment including a careful myofascial examination and spinal mobility evaluation are techniques that are integral to understanding these cases.
- There are many treatment modalities available, and generally, the multimodal approach, including integrative therapy, improves the overall outcome.

INTRODUCTION

Cervical pain and/or dysfunction is often a frustrating condition for horse owners as well as the veterinarian evaluating or managing the case. Frequently, conventional medicine feels inadequate diagnostically and therapeutically. It is not uncommon for owners of these cases to seek out evaluation by veterinarians with additional training in integrative medicine after they feel conventional therapies have not been successful. Understanding the myofascial system, and the information that is attainable through a thorough myofascial and spinal mobility examination, is extremely valuable in giving a better understanding of the complexity of each case of cervical pain and dysfunction. Training in integrative therapies often-times gives the practitioner skills in evaluation that are not commonly taught through conventional training.

After systematically going through all of the steps of a thorough evaluation, which includes carefully listening to the history, understanding behavioral changes associated with the horse, the myofascial, mobility, and motion examinations, and associated diagnostic imaging, then a thorough therapeutic plan can be made. Therapy that includes integrative medicine allows the practitioner many more options than what is available through conventional medicine alone. Integrative medicine is safe, and many times very effective in managing a horse with cervical pain and dysfunction. If the practitioner finds this first-tiered approach is not enough, more therapies may be

The author has nothing to disclose.
Equine Sports Medicine and Rehabilitation, Orthopedic Research Center, C. Wayne McIlwraith Translational Medicine Institute, Department of Clinical Sciences, Colorado State University, 2350 Research Boulevard, Fort Collins, CO 80526, USA
E-mail address: Melinda.story@colostate.edu

layered on, as a multimodal approach, combining integrative and conventional medicine. This method is frequently very beneficial leading to a comfortable, functional horse, and a satisfied owner.

HISTORY

Gathering a thorough history is always a critical first step when evaluating a patient, particularly when there are behavioral issues at hand.[1,2] In some cases of cervical pain and dysfunction, there may be a history of overt injury such as a trailer accident or a fall. However, frequently there may not be any known inciting cause or specific timeline; these cases may be more insidious in nature, showing a gradual decline in performance due to neck stiffness and pain. As the horse is continually asked to perform the exercises that cause discomfort, the resistance may escalate. Ultimately, these horses may progress to the point of dangerous behavior resulting in injury of the horse and/or the rider. In one case series describing dangerous behavior in performance horses, there was a common history of recent purchase,[3] and there is speculation that extended travel and relocation may exacerbate cervical pain and dysfunction. When gathering historical information, knowledge of prior treatments (including the degree of improvement and length of time of improvement) is also important information to note. It has been shown that diagnostic analgesia in horses exhibiting pain behavior under saddle will improve the behavior scores with the resolution of the lameness.[4] Many times the behavior is not linked as easily to pain from a lameness, and instead, the owners will notice subtle changes in the horse, how they respond to routines such as grooming and tacking up, and their facial expressions while standing in the stall.[5] Listen to these comments as they may be very strong signs that the horse is in fact experiencing pain, which should then lead to a very thorough and systematic approach to the assessment of the horse.

ASSESSMENT

Evaluating a horse for cervical pain and dysfunction may seem complicated. However, when using a systematic approach; starting with a visual exam, followed by a thorough myofascial examination, assessing for spinal mobility, and finally watching the horse in motion, the process will become more straightforward and lead to a better understanding of these difficult cases.

The visual examination is a crucial element to begin the examination process. As stated above, the owners will often report observations indicating the horse may be exhibiting pain behavior. It is beneficial for the clinician to evaluate the horse in the home environment to pick up on subtle behavioral signs. The excitement or stress of the new environment at a clinic or hospital may override signs of pain and discomfort. However, observing the horse in the stall gives immediate indicators of comfort and should not be overlooked. Starting with facial expressions,[5] there are signs of pain that can be quickly evident. A change in position of the eyes, ears, and mouth is very easy to assess and serves as an indicator of the level of discomfort.[6] In addition, looking at the neck position and if the horse has an antalgic stance may be indicative of pain or discomfort. If the horse shows an inability to stand squarely while relaxing in the stall (shifting weight from forelimbs to hindlimbs, or shifting from side to side), or if one limb is rested out in front of the other, this is frequently noted as a sign of pain (**Fig. 1**). Watching the horse in the stall for positioning and desire to engage with humans may also help in identifying pain. If the horse is standing in the back of the stall and does not want to engage when a person walks up, or if they hold the neck stretched out in a rigid and guarded fashion when they turn to look toward the stall door, this may also

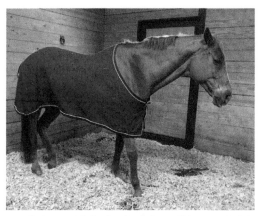

Fig. 1. The horse is standing toward the back of the stall in an antalgic stance, disengaged with the surroundings. Note the front limbs are not in a square stance, the muzzle is tight, and the ears are flat.

indicate the horse is uncomfortable. Abnormal sweat patterns, a subtle trembling of the leg, or an over-at-the-knee posture may be secondary to nerve dysfunction and many times are indications of abnormalities associated with the cervical region. When any of these signs are noted, further evaluation of the cervical spine is indicated.

Once the horse has been led out of the stall, then further visual and digital palpation examinations may ensue. Look for muscle symmetry, not only from side to side, but also front to back. In a horse with a muscular and symmetric hind quarter, with a thin, under-muscled neck, this may be a sign of cervical pain and dysfunction[7] and warrants further evaluation. Digital palpation begins with superficial palpation of the skin and fascia, monitoring for heat or cool areas, and for tone or signs of tightness of the fascia. There should not be any negative reaction from the horse as the fascia glides across the underlying muscles. Palpation moves deeper into the muscles, assessing for tone and texture and evaluating for trigger points (painful, tight bands within the muscle tissue). In the authors opinion, acupuncture points such as LI-18 (cranial) and ST-10 (caudal) in the brachiocephalicus may be found to be reactive in horses protecting their neck or associated with front limb lameness. Additional acupuncture points commonly noted by the author to be reactive in horses with caudal cervical pain are LI-16, LI-17, and BL-13 and BL-10, while SI-16, and TH-16 may be reactive in the cranial region. Lastly, in the static examination, look for an avoidance response to deep palpation of the cervical articular process joints and the transverse processes. This static examination, carried out systematically from both sides of the horse, starting with the most superficial tissues and carefully evaluating each tissue type going deeply to the level of the bone structure and articular process joints, will decrease the risk of missing important indicators of pain and/or dysfunction of the cervical spine.

After the static examination has been completed, then spinal mobility may be assessed. When testing for normal mobility of the cervical spine, both passive and active movements are used to investigate joint and soft-tissue movement without muscle activation (passive), and when the patient initiates the motion (active).[8] Lateral bending is performed being careful that the eyes stay horizontal as the horse moves the neck to each side (**Fig. 2**). Flexion and extension motion is also assessed and all movements are evaluated for range of motion and the ease in which the horse moves through the exercises. In horses with cervical pain and dysfunction, any or all of these exercises may be difficult and result in avoidance behavior. In some horses the behavior may be as simple as just not doing the exercise, in horses experiencing more discomfort, the reaction may be very abrupt and even dangerous if the practitioner tries to force mobility.

The final step of a thorough evaluation is watching the horse in motion. Both the musculoskeletal and neurologic systems should be thoroughly assessed. Horses with cervical pain and dysfunction may have very subtle gait abnormalities that often require watching the horse in hand at the walk and trot as well as lunging at the walk, trot, and canter. Additional information may be gained from evaluation with tack on, and if safe, with a rider. Routine lameness and neurologic deficits, including weakness, ataxia, and stumbling are noted. Cervical disease should be considered in horses with a front limb lameness that is not able to be isolated to the appendicular skeleton with a complete blocking evaluation. Some horses may also show signs related to cervical pain and dysfunction in how they use their body in motion. Perhaps they hold the head and neck stiff and in abnormal posture, they may adapt the flight pattern of a forelimb, or have a "hoping-like" motion.[9,10] Horses may only show behavioral changes in that they may toss their head, show difficulty to hold the head straight and accept contact with the bit, or they may not want to move forward and become quite resistant when asked, to the point of abruptly stopping, refusing to move and perhaps rearing and becoming dangerous to themselves and rider.

DIAGNOSTIC IMAGING

Diagnostic imaging of the cervical spine adds important information to our understanding of cervical pain and dysfunction. However, it is important to acknowledge that there are limitations to all of the modalities utilized. Radiographs are the most commonly used imaging modality and serve as a good baseline screening tool; however, clinical significance of the findings must be well correlated.[11] A complete series of radiographs are necessary to gain as much information as possible. This includes lateral-lateral radiographs from the level of the occiput to the first thoracic (T1)

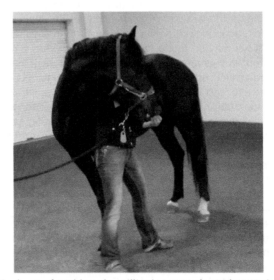

Fig. 2. The horse looks comfortable as he willingly moves through a cervical lateral bending exercise. The eyes are horizontal, the body square, and no avoidance is noted in this active-assisted movement.

vertebrae if the size of the horse does not preclude beam penetration. In addition, oblique radiographs are becoming much more commonly evaluated to gain an understanding of laterality of noted lesions. It is recommended to seek referral if a complete series is not possible with field radiograph equipment to decrease the potential for misinterpretation from a non-diagnostic study.

Frequently utilized in combination with radiographs, ultrasound imaging of the cervical spine will allow the practitioner to further assess the APJ margins, joint capsules, and regional soft tissues. Again, a complete examination is performed from the level of the occiput to the last visible articulation, most commonly C7-T1.[12]

Nuclear scintigraphy, although commonly used to aid in the diagnosis of lameness or poor performance in the appendicular skeleton, is not as beneficial in the axial skeleton and may produce false-positive results when used for imaging the cervical spine.[13] Keep in mind that false-negative results may also occur because of the overlying musculature and scapular shielding.[13] If there is a negative result when using nuclear scintigraphy, it only means there is not active bone turnover. It is not interpreted to mean there is not pain or dysfunction coming from the cervical region.[14]

Three-dimensional imaging is becoming the modality of choice when facing complicated cases with signs of neck pain and stiffness. These modalities include computed tomography (CT), and CT myelography. MRI would allow for a more thorough evaluation of the soft tissues, including nervous tissue; however, it is not possible to image the caudal cervical spine in an adult horse[9] and will therefore not be discussed further. CT examination allows for a detailed evaluation of osseous abnormalities and implications to the surrounding soft-tissue structures. More thorough answers for the owners, and treatment options more appropriately targeted at the tissue or structure of concern, will be more widely available as more hospitals offer the ability for evaluation of the cervical spine with advanced imaging.

PRIMARY TREATMENTS

Integrative medicine is commonly used as a first-line treatment for horses experiencing varying levels of cervical pain and dysfunction. When working through these cases, it is important to identify the primary goals of treatment. Pain modulation is generally the first and most important component to consider. It has been suggested that a subset of horses presenting for behavioral concerns may be experiencing neuropathic pain.[3] When this is the case, routine medications and treatments targeted primarily at inflammation will not be as effective as desired. There are a multitude of integrative therapies that may be utilized to modulate pain. This author incorporates acupuncture routinely in horses showing signs of neck pain and stiffness. There is a great diagnostic value (understanding the myofascial examination) and therapeutic value (dry needle, acupressure, aquapuncture, and electrical stimulation) when implementing acupuncture in these cases. However, it is also important to recognize that in a horse in a neuropathic pain state, they may be experiencing allodynia and/or hyperalgesia and stimulation of the nervous system through acupuncture may be too much for the horse to accept. In these instances, other integrative options may be considered to maintain a safe experience for the veterinarian and owner/handler of the horse. In addition to electroacupuncture, other electrotherapies such as transcutaneous nerve stimulation (TENS) and pulsed electromagnetic field therapy (PEMF) may be utilized for pain modulation. LASER therapy and extracorporeal shockwave therapy (ESWT) are also frequently performed in cases presenting for cervical pain and dysfunction (**Fig. 3**). In addition to decreasing pain, ESWT may be used to improve myofascial pain and restricted mobility in horses as has been shown in humans.[15] Improving mobility is another important goal for managing horses experiencing pain and stiffness in the cervical spine. Chiropractic care is routinely performed to improve stiffness. In some cases, the horse is too reactive, or perhaps there is segmental instability that would deem chiropractic an unsafe treatment. Improving stiffness in these horses is primarily through therapeutic exercises. The goal of these exercises is to improve flexibility and strength.[16]

In addition to these physical medicine techniques, supporting the body through good nutrition is a critical component of successful management. Understanding how the diet and exercise program of each horse influences the metabolic status is important. Some horses, presenting for behavioral challenges that seem connected to the cervical spine, may have underlying myopathies such as polysaccharide storage myopathy and vitamin E-related myopathies. These conditions are particularly susceptible to exacerbation of clinical signs based on the nutritional status of the horse. Even when there is not an underlying muscle or vitamin issue of concern, improving the comfort and function of many cases may be improved with careful evaluation of the diet. It is well recognized that natural healing may be impacted through herbal and nutritional supplementation. It is advised to seek out those with a thorough understanding of these methods to avoid over-supplementation and potentially dangerous cross-reactions of supplements.

SECONDARY TREATMENTS

Multimodal therapy is often indicated in the more complicated cases. Frequently medications may be utilized in addition to the therapies discussed above. There may be indications for systemic use, local administration, or both. If there is a clinically significant inflammatory component to the neck pain such as in an acute injury, or if there are ongoing chronic inflammatory conditions such as osteoarthritis, steroid, and nonsteroidal anti-inflammatory medications may be warranted. These may include medications such as prednisolone, phenylbutazone, or flunixin meglumine. In the author's opinion, firocoxib is often not effective in managing cases of cervical pain and dysfunction. Medications for muscle relaxation such as methocarbamol may also be indicated in specific circumstances, but are not commonly utilized in the majority of cases. Pain medications that may target more of a neuropathic pain state may be indicated in some horses. Gabapentin has been used in veterinary patients[17] and in human medicine[18] to address neuropathic pain states and has been used with some success in horses with behavioral concerns stemming from chronic pain.

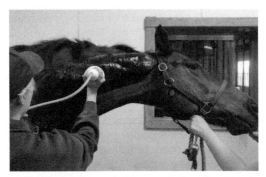

Fig. 3. Extracorporeal shockwave therapy of the cervical region of an unsedated horse. The author uses shockwave therapy to reduce muscle tension, treat muscle or ligament injuries, and to help with, pain modulation from articular process joint osteoarthritis. This modality may be effectively used in horses where acupuncture is deemed unsafe.

In addition to systemic medications, local therapies may also be warranted. In horses experiencing neck pain and stiffness, efforts to define where the pain is coming from certainly will improve the treatment efficacy. When articular process joints are involved, intra-articular (IA), ultrasound-guided therapy is often indicated. Similar to IA therapy of the appendicular skeleton, treatment with corticosteroids, Hyaluronic acid, and biologic therapies may all be considered as viable treatment options.[14]

TERTIARY TREATMENTS

Infrequently, surgical intervention may be necessary to manage these horses. Although there are arthroscopic techniques previously described for the cervical articular process joints,[19-21] they did not show a great success. A more recent report gives more encouraging outcomes and warrants considering arthroscopy at C5-C6 or C6-C7 in select cases.[22] Surgical stabilization of the cervical spine may improve the outcome in young, as well as in older horses with cervical vertebral stenotic myopathy.[23] Stabilization techniques may also be considered in select horses displaying behavioral abnormalities related to cervical pain and dysfunction.

SUMMARY

Horses experiencing cervical pain and dysfunction are challenging. However, when approached in a systematic way, many times the outcomes are quite rewarding. Listening carefully to the history is a critical starting point. Performing a very thorough physical examination is of paramount importance and must include a visual, myofascial, mobility, and motion evaluation to best understand the condition of the horse. Utilizing multiple imaging modalities is frequently helpful and must be correlated to the clinical picture. There are multiple considerations when developing a treatment plan. Integrative therapies are often used as stand-alone therapies, or along with other treatments. Although there are cases that are refractory to all applied treatments, in many instances improvements in the condition and successful management of horses with varying levels of cervical pain and dysfunction is possible.

CLINICS CARE POINTS

- Applying integrative training allows the practitioner to have added insight to the source of cervical pain and dysfunction.
- There are multiple integrative therapies that may be used for pain modulation in cases of cervical pain and dysfuntion.
- In horses experiencing allodynia and/or hyperalgesia, therapies such as acupuncture should be used with caution.

REFERENCES

1. Dyson S, Berger J, Ellis AD, et al. Development of an ethogram for a pain scoring system in ridden horses and its application to determine the presence of musculoskeletal pain. J Vet Behav 2018;23:47–57.
2. Kjaerulff LNR, Lindegaard C. Performance and rideability issues in horses as a manifestation of pain: a review of differential diagnosis and diagnostic approach. Equine Vet Ed 2020;34:103–12.

3. Story MR, Nout-Lomas YS, Aboellail TA, et al. Dangerous behavior and intractable axial skeletal pain in performance horses: a possible role for ganglioneuritis (14 Cases; 2014-2019). Front Vet Sci 2021;8:734218.

4. Dyson S, Van Dijk J. Application of a ridden horse ethogram to video recordings of 21 horses before and after diagnostic analgesia: Reduction in behaviour scores. Equine Vet 2020;32:104–11.

5. Dalla Costa E, Minero M, Lebelt D, et al. Development of the Horse Grimace Scale (HGS) as a pain assessment tool in horses undergoing routine castration. PLoS One 2014;9(3):e92281.

6. Gleerup KB, Forkman B, Lindegaard C, et al. An equine pain face. Vet Anaesth Analg 2015;42(1):103–14.

7. Koenig JB, Westlund A, Nykamp S, et al. Case-control comparison of cervical spine radiographs from horses with a clinical diagnosis of cervical facet disease with normal horses. J Eq Vet Sci 2020;92:1–6.

8. Haussler KK. Joint mobilization and manipulation for the equine athlete. Vet Clin North Am Equine Pract 2016;32(1):87–101.

9. Dyson S. Unexplained forelimb lameness possibly assoiciated with radiculopathy. Equine Vet Ed 2020;32:92–103.

10. Dyson S, Rasotto R. Idiopathic hopping-like forelimb lameness syndrome in ridden horses: 46 horses (2002-2014). Equine Vet 2016;28(1):30–9.

11. Down SS, Henson FM. Radiographic retrospective study of the caudal cervical articular process joints in the horse. Equine Vet J 2009;41(6):518–24.

12. Selberg K, Barrett M. Imaging of the equine neck. AAEP 2016;34–41, 360 proceedings.

13. Dyson SJ. Lesions of the equine neck resulting in lameness or poor performance. Vet Clin North Am Equine Pract 2011;27(3):417–37.

14. Story MR, Haussler KK, Nout-Lomas YS, et al. Equine cervical pain and dysfunction: pathology, diagnosis and treatment. Animals (Basel) 2021;11(2). https://doi.org/10.3390/ani11020422.

15. Jeon JH, Jung YJ, Lee JY, et al. The effect of extracorporeal shock wave therapy on myofascial pain syndrome. Ann Rehabil Med 2012;36(5):665–74.

16. Clayton HM, Kaiser LJ, Lavagnino M, et al. Dynamic mobilisations in cervical flexion: Effects on intervertebral angulations. Equine Vet J Suppl 2010;(38):688–94.

17. Adrian D, Papich M, Baynes R, et al. Chronic maladaptive pain in cats: a review of current and future drug treatment options. Vet J 2017;230:52–61.

18. Finnerup NB, Attal N, Haroutounian S, et al. Pharmacotherapy for neuropathic pain in adults: a systematic review and meta-analysis. Lancet Neurol 2015;14(2):162–73.

19. Perez-Nogues M, Vaughan B, Phillips KL, et al. Evaluation of the caudal cervical articular process joints by using a needle arthroscope in standing horses. Vet Surg 2020;49(3):463–71.

20. Pepe M, Angelone M, Gialletti R, et al. Arthroscopic anatomy of the equine cervical articular process joints. Equine Vet J 2014;46(3):345–51.

21. Tucker RPR, Dixon JJ, Muir CF, et al. Arthroscopic treatment for cervical articular process joint osteochondrosis in a Thoroughbred horse. Equine Vet Ed 2018;30:116–21.

22. Schulze N, Ehrle A, Beckmann I, et al. Arthroscopic removal of osteochondral fragments of the cervical articular process joints in three horses. Vet Surg 2021. https://doi.org/10.1111/vsu.13681.

23. Anderson J. Wobbler surgery: what is the evidence? Equine Vet Ed 2020;32(3):166–8.

Clinical Application of Myofascial Therapy in Horses

Tuulia Luomala, PT

KEYWORDS

- Fascia • Myofascial treatment • Myofascial pain • Densification • Dysfunction

KEY POINTS

- The fascial system is a complex, three-dimensional network that envelops and interconnects all tissues and structures.
- Fascia functions in proprioception, force transmission, and shock absorption.
- Myofascial tissues can be a clinically significant source of a pain.
- Fascial tissues can be treated with superficial and deep myofascial techniques.

 Video content accompanies this article at http://www.vetequine.theclinics. com.

INTRODUCTION

Fascia forms a complex three-dimensional network that surrounds and forms the structural properties of all tissues within the body. Myofascial tissues are critical both for support and movement. As we push horses to extreme limits of athletic performance, many horses are presented with clinical signs of myofascial pain and dysfunctions. Specific techniques can be used to diagnose and treatment myofascial issues in horses.

THE FASCIAL SYSTEM

Fascia consists of different types of connective tissue that unites, protects, encloses, and separates body regions or tissues. Fascia consists of combinations of varying composition, density, forms, and regularities, for example, loose, dense, regular, and irregular connective tissue.[1] The fascial system is complex with respect to its architecture and function. The fascial system forms a three-dimensional continuum of

Figures and videos: Mika Pihlman.
MT-Physio Oy, Hakkarintie 5, Lempäälä 37550, Finland
E-mail address: tuulia.luomala@gmail.com

collagen fibers that can be organized into loose or dense, irregular or regular tissue layers because it permeates throughout the body.[2]

The fascial system includes the following:

- Superficial fascia
- Deep fascia
- Fibroadipose tissue
- Neurovascular sheaths and epineurium
- Joint capsules, ligaments, and tendons
- Periosteum and entheses
- Myofascial expansions (connections from muscles and tendons inserting into deep fascia)
- Retinacula and septa
- Intermuscular and intramuscular structures
- Plural and peritoneal linings
- Visceral coverings and mesenteric attachments

Connective tissue persists at the cellular, to tissue, to organ levels within the body. Fascia varies widely in its structure from thin endomysium surrounding the muscle cell, to thicker perimysium constraining muscle fibers, and to robust epimysium encapsulating the muscle belly itself (**Fig. 1**). Intermuscular septa and tendons are formed by myofascial expansions. Deep fascia provides anchorage for the superficial fascia and overlying dermis and skin (**Fig. 2**). The fascial system that surrounds and provides support for the internal organs also has origins from the deep fascia. As an example, the epimysium of the diaphragm and abdominal wall is continuous with the fibrous capsule of the liver via ligamentous connections (eg, triangular and falciform ligaments, respectively, **Fig. 3**).[2]

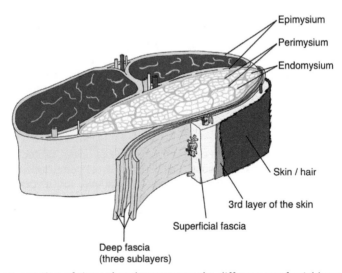

Fig. 1. A cross-section of tissue that demonstrates the different myofascial layers from the skin (epidermis, dermis, and third layer of the skin*), to superficial fascia, to deep fascia, and then intermuscular fascia. *Deeper dense parallel collagen layer (accessory Cordovan layer), which is only present in horses compared with humans and dogs (Waqas A. et al., 2019). (*Courtesy of* Mika Pihlman.)

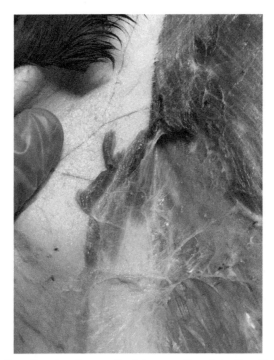

Fig. 2. Anatomic dissection showing myofascial connections from the skin to the superficial fascia and cutaneous trunci. Under the cutaneous trunci lay deep adipose and loose connective tissue connected to deep fascia.

At the Cellular Level

Fibroblasts are the most common cell type in the connective tissue. Fibroblasts have high building and repairing capacity, and the main function of these cells is to maintain the structural integrity of the connective tissue by secreting collagen and elastic fibers. Fibroblasts react to tension by increasing collagen synthesis and hereby strengthening the area.[3,4]

At the Fiber Level

Collagen is the most abundant structural protein in the body making up to 35% of the whole-body protein mass. The arrangement of the collagen fibers can be parallel or nonparallel. The arrangements are reflections of the tension and compression applied to the tissue. Collagen is responsible for the force transmission and stability of the body parts. Currently, there are 28 different recognized types of collagen.[5] At the fiber level, elastin and reticular fibers also intermingle with the collagen fibers to increase the elasticity of connective tissue. In general, an increased collagen content produces more resistance to tension and increased elastin provides more elasticity.[3]

At the Tissue Level

Fascia is divided in the 2 major groups characterized as loose or dense connective tissue. Loose connective tissue is irregular, and its main function is to support movement between different structures or tissue layers and, at the same time, restrict excessive motion. Loose connective tissue has a high concentration of hyaluronan, which

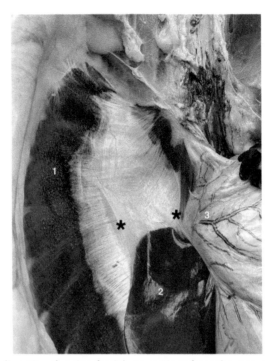

Fig. 3. Anatomic dissection showing fascial connections from the stomach and the liver toward the diaphragm. Connections are marked with *asterisks.* (1) Diaphragm. (2) Liver. (3) Stomach.

contributes to its hydration with viscous and gel-like properties. Dense connective tissue includes deep fascia, aponeurosis, ligament, tendons, and joint capsules. The major role of dense connective tissue is to transmit and absorb forces (**Fig. 4**).[6,7]

HOW IS FASCIA ORGANIZED?

Fascia can be defined and illustrated many ways. Tissue layer and compartmental models are useful to visualize the complex architecture of the fascial system.

Tissue Layer Model

In the layer model, the connective tissue layers include superficial fascia under the skin, then deep adipose tissue, deep fascia, and then muscles and organs enclosed within their own capsules (eg, pericardium of the heart and epimysium of the muscle). In the trunk region, the cutaneous trunci muscle is enclosed by the superficial fascia. In the limbs, superficial and deep fascias are fused tightly together and adipose tissue is almost absent (**Fig. 5**). Although the layer model is a simplified way of organizing the fascial layers, it gives an idea of the three-dimensional continuum forming interconnected tissue layers from the surface to deeper regions of the body.[8]

Compartmental Model

In the compartmental model, fascial connections from different layers coalesce and surround muscle groups within the deeper parts of the body (eg, flexor and extensor compartment of the thoracic limb; **Fig. 6**). Skin surrounds the whole limb and the

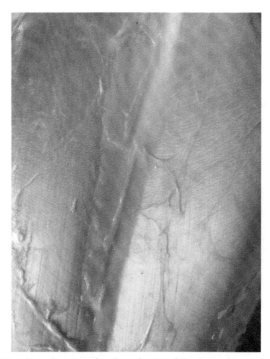

Fig. 4. Anatomic dissection showing the deep fascia of the lateral scapular region. The scapular spine is evident in the middle of the image between the supraspinatus and infraspinatus muscles that are covered with deep fascia.

underlying superficial and deep fascia form sock-like coverings within the limb and create strong attachments to the bone, where dense septa are created between the flexor and extensor compartments. In the area of the trunk, epaxial and hypaxial muscles are surrounded within fascial compartments that attach to the transversus processes. Visceral fascia also forms connections with the myofascial system to create a fascial continuum from inside to outside regions of the body (eg, peritoneal and plural cavities).

Functionally fascia is participating to the shock absorption, proprioception, and force transmission. Because fascia is creating separation, support, frame and connection, mobility and stability are important features of this intriguing tissue.[2]

MYOFASCIAL DYSFUNCTION

The fascial system is organized in several layers and sublayers in multidirectional orientations (**Fig. 7**). When the horse is moving, this system provides mobility and stability between different structures (ie, myofascia, articular, neural, and vascular components). Loose connective tissue plays a key role in the movement between the different tissue layers, whereas dense connective tissue provides structural support and stability for the body.

Factors that cause changes in fascial viscosity within the myofascial system have been studied more closely. Viscoelastic changes have been visualized between the

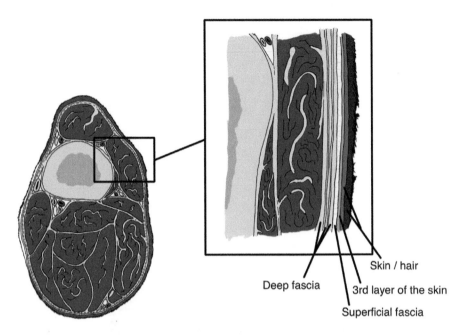

Skin / hair

Deep fascia

3rd layer of the skin

Superficial fascia

Horse, right thoracic limb

Fig. 5. A cross-section of the equine forelimb. Under the skin lays superficial fascia. The deep fascia is tightly adhered to the superficial fascia. The fascial system formed by the epimysium and perimysium are also visible in this sagittal section. (*Courtesy of* Mika Pihlman.)

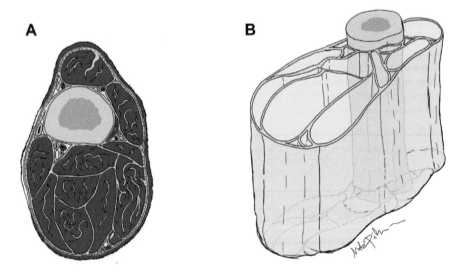

Horse, right thoracic limb

Fig. 6. A cross-section of the equine forelimb at the level of the radius (*A*) reveals myofascial connections from the surface to the deeper portion of the body. Flexor and extensor compartments are highlighted in B, where the actin and myosin has been removed and the supporting fascial structures extend from the surface to the radius. (*Courtesy of* Mika Pihlman.)

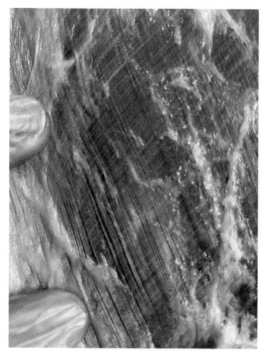

Fig. 7. Anatomic dissection showing how collagen fibers form a criss-cross orientation on surface of the muscle belly.

deep fascial layers with ultrasonography and elastography.[9] Myofascial dysfunction has also been documented with $T_{1\rho}$-mapping with a reported decreased capacity of hyaluronan to bind water.[10]

Inflammatory process can reduce the local pH of tissues because more acidic condition may contribute to changes in the viscosity of hyaluronan. This can then reduce the mobility of the myofascial system.[11]

Myofascial dysfunctions can be categorized into 3 different types (**Fig. 8**):

- *Densification* is a viscoelastic change within the loose connective tissue, which can be treated within few minutes with mechanical friction. Densification can also affect the loose connective tissue between the deep fascial layers. Densification does not cause histologic changes within the dense connective tissue. Densification is formed because of overuse, misuse, or disuse of fascial tissues. It can be present also after trauma or chronic, repetitive use injuries.
- *Adhesions* are characterized by changes in the loose and dense connective tissue. Adhesions can be formed after trauma or surgical procedures through the early tissue healing phases. Collagen fibers are formed and orientating in lines of tension or where tissues are reinforced. Adhesions can be reduced and overall viscosity of the tissue may be improved but dense or extensive adhesions (ie, scar tissue) is difficult to change.
- *Fibrosis* is caused by histologic changes within the dense connective tissue. Fibrosis can be formed due to long-term stress or tissue inflammation. Fibrosis

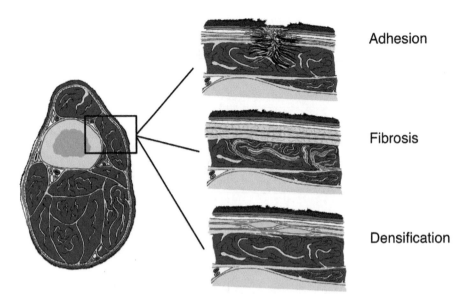

Fig. 8. A cross-section of tissue that demonstrates adhesions, fibrosis, and densification. Adhesion is characterized by misalignment of collagen fibers that forms a mesh that penetrates all tissue layers (ie, scar). Fibrosis occurs when dense connective tissue becomes thickened and collagen type I is changing to collagen type III. Densification occurs between the dense connective tissue layers and may alter the viscoelasticity of the overlying loose connective tissue. (*Courtesy of* Mika Pihlman.)

causes permanent changes within the connective tissue where treatment may improve the overall tissue elasticity but the fibrosis itself cannot be changed.

Myofascial dysfunction can be caused by overuse, disuse, misuse, or trauma. Myofascial dysfunction may be localized to one region of the body and then can be compensated distant to the initial site of injury.[12]

HOW TO PALPATE SUPERFICIAL AND DEEP MYOFASCIAL STRUCTURES?

Observing the hair and skin can provide a first glance to a horse's myofascial system. Visual signs include swelling, muscle atrophy, asymmetries, and tensioned areas within the myofascial tissue. The skin and underlying dermis are characterized by cleavage lines, which provide insights into fascial patterns, especially when attempting to close open wounds or when making surgical incisions.[13] It is important to recognize regional differences in skin and dermal mobility while performing superficial palpation. Different areas of the body have different skin and superficial fascial movements.

Superficial palpation is applied with a light touch (Video 1). The skin and superficial fascia can be moved in all directions. With superficial palpation, it is possible to sense changes in tension or resistance within the skin, superficial and deep fascia. It is possible to assess fascial restrictions within deeper tissues by pulling or applying tension to the skin and superficial fascia.

Deep soft tissue palpation has a focus more on evaluation of the deep fascia and muscles bellies (Video 2). The applied pressure is more localized and firmer, and the induced displacement or movement of the underlying tissue is smaller than when applying superficial palpation. With deep palpation, it is possible to detect tension within the muscles and localize adhesions and fibrosis related to dysfunction of the deep fascia (Video 3).

HOW TO TREAT SUPERFICIAL AND DEEP MYOFASCIAL STRUCTURES?

To understand effects of the myofascial techniques, we first need to be familiar with the mechanoreceptors of the body. These specialized receptors (eg, free nerve endings, Vater and Pacinian corpuscles, Ruffini corpuscles, Meissner corpuscles) are designed to sense changes in tension, pressure, vibration, and shearing forces. The muscle spindles and Golgi tendon organs (GTO) are also relaying information about muscle length and tension from the periphery to the central nervous system. Increased tension within the intramuscular fascia and collagen fibers surrounding the GTOs reflexively induces muscle relaxation. Because the skin, superficial and deep fascia are richly innervated with a multitude of differing fascial receptors, light touch or firmer palpation may both be equally effective treatment options, depending on the condition of the underlying tissue.[14]

Myofascial receptors react to different types of stimuli where Pacinian corpuscles are activated by rapid oscillations and rhythmic movements, whereas Ruffini nerve endings are stimulated by slower shearing forces. Ruffini nerve endings also influence the parasympathetic nervous system in that slower myofascial techniques often induce relaxation within the body.

Myofascial treatment techniques:

- *Slow gliding* is often used to induce relaxation (Videos 4 and 5). The applied technique takes time because the therapist needs to progress slowly and let the underlying tissues respond to the slow, superficial movements.
- *Light touch* applied along the lines of myofascial tension is useful in very painful situations (Video 6). Light touch is also useful when a horse is very nervous or anxious. These techniques are typically very relaxing and soothing (Video 7).
- *Cross-fiber friction massage* is typically quite fast and applied rhythmically (Videos 8 and 9). The technique can be applied rapidly while mechanical friction begins to loosen myofascial tissues within 2 to 3 minutes per tensional area. Once the underlying tissue starts to relax, the applied pressure is applied faster and extended from one affected area to the next. Cross-fiber friction massage can be applied for both relaxation and activation purposes.
- *Ischemic compression* is typically applied when underlying myofascial tissue is under substantial tension and local pain responses (eg, active trigger point) are noted when deep pressure is applied to the affected tissue (Video 10).

Myofascial treatment variables (Video 11):

- *Depth* of the applied treatment is varying according to the type of myofascial dysfunction and tolerance of the individual horse. Myofascial dysfunction can be localized to the superficial or deeper tissue layers and detailed palpation can localize the depth of the needed treatment technique.
- *Direction* of the applied technique is based on the individual patient due to compensation patterns created by tension and adhesions or fibrosis. Some directions of fascial mobility may be good (eg, craniocaudal), whereas, at the same time, other directions (ie, mediolateral) may be dysfunctional, even within the same area of the body.

- *Speed* is defined by the desired therapeutic outcome. Slower techniques are often more relaxing and faster techniques are activating within the myofascial tissues.
- *Rhythm* of the treatment is individually based. Some horses relax better with more rhythmic techniques, and some horses may need more static pressure to produce the desired therapeutic effects.
- *Angle* of the applied treatment depends on the body area treated. Perpendicular forces are often firmer and stronger, compared with shearing or gliding techniques (Video 12).

Myofascial treatments are focusing to improve viscoelasticity, fluid dynamics, and movement between different fascial structures.[9]

Myofascial treatment goals are as follows:

- Patient relaxation
- Reduce pain
- Reduce tension within myofascial structures
- Increase the joint and spinal mobility
- Improve proprioception and body awareness
- Enhance muscle recruitment and improve motor control
- Improve tissue healing and recovery after trauma or surgical procedures

MYOFASCIAL PAIN

Can fascia be a source of pain? Based on the current body of scientific evidence, it seems that pain may induce changes in fascial thickness, mobility, viscoelasticity, and associated neurotransmitters and endocannabinoid receptors.[10,15] Although many studies about the interaction between fascia and pain syndromes have been conducted in humans and rats, studies are needed in horses to understand the difference between various species.

Human subjects experiencing back pain have thicker fascia and decreased mobility between the thoracolumbar fascial layers.[16] In humans with chronic neck pain, an increase in fascial thickness of the sternocleidomastoid muscle has been reported.[17] The thoracolumbar fascia is reported to be the most pain-sensitive tissue within the human back.[18] Hypertonic saline injections into the skin, fascia, and muscle produced different sensation with fascial pain being described as agonizing, exhausting, and heavy.[18]

Thoracolumbar fascia and its innervation have been reported in humans and rats.[19] Inflamed fascia has increased concentrations of calcitonin gene-related peptide and substance P, which support the hypothesis that free nerve endings function as nociceptors and that the thoracolumbar fascia as a primary source of pain.[19] Myofascial pain can also affect hormonal mechanisms and associated endocannabinoid receptors 1 and 2 within the deep fascia, which are involved in pain modulation.[20] Recent studies support the hypothesis that myofascial pain can be relieved with myofascial treatments. For example, C tactile fibers have been detected within the skin, which react to gentle touch by secreting oxytocin and reinforce the perceived value of physical contact and social interaction.[21]

Tools used to assess myofascial pain include the following:

- Equine grimace scale—pinned ears
- Behavioral changes—fear responses

- Provocation tests—passive soft tissue movement
- Palpation—heat, swelling, dysfunction in the myofascial tissue such as densification or muscular tightness

---

The horse can reflect the mental stress of the rider. Horses can even distinguish positive and negative human facial expression in a photograph. A facial action coding system was used to analyze horses' responses to viewing a positive or negative human face where it was found that horses had higher heart rates when shown a picture of a negative human face, compared with a positive human face.[22] There are 17 defined facial expression defined in horses (humans have 27).[23]

CLINICAL CASE EXAMPLES

Case 1. A 12-year-old Holsteiner mare was purchased by here current owner in 2020 and they have been competing in eventing together since. At the clinical presentation at that time, the mare had displayed a lot of pain signals, which included pinned ears, anxiety when saddling, angry when brushing the abdominal area, swishing the tail, and lack of trust toward people. The owner complained that the horse seemed crooked, the fascia over the left shoulder and scapular area was tight, and the right pelvic limb was weak. Propulsion was inadequate, and the horse was not jumping straight.

Assessment of the horse verified the owner's concerns. The superficial fascia over the left scapula and shoulder joint area seemed restricted, movement of the left thoracic limb was limited in protraction and retraction, and internal–external rotation of the forelimb was limited. Myofascial palpation identified tension in the superficial pectoral area and over the lateral scapula. Palpation of lower cervical area revealed pain and tension in the brachiocephalicus and cervical trapezius muscles.

Myofascial treatment of the affected areas provided relief of the clinical signs with continued treatment provided during the last 2 years. At this moment, the horse and the rider are competing internationally in eventing. Propulsion of the pelvic limbs is equal, the horse is overall stronger, and the left thoracic limb can now move freely. However, when the horse tires, prior maladaptive movement patterns recur. Fortunately, periodic myofascial treatment has quickly resolved any clinical complaints. The owner is satisfied with the horse's performance, and the horse has been progressively improving during the last 2 years without any further injuries.

Case 2. A 14-year-old Finnish mare has poor conformation of the topline and inadequate activation of the pectoral and abdominal muscles. At the age of 8 years, she developed chronic carpal canal inflammation within both thoracic limbs, which was treated surgically when the mare was 10 year old. Postoperatively, myofascial treatments played a crucial role in her rehabilitation. Treatment was focused on the surgical incision sites and extended outward to include the thoracic limb. The mare consistently had tension in the biceps brachii, superficial pectoral, and trapezius muscles. Exercises have focused on improving the activation of the pectoral and abdominal muscles and pelvic limb impulsion. She has improved to compete at the national level in dressage and is currently performing well without pain or signs of thoracic lameness.

SUGGESTIONS FOR THE MYOFASCIAL TREATMENT PLAN

Myofascial dysfunction and pain can be detected with observation, palpation, and active and passive motion testing. Chronic myofascial dysfunction can create compensational patterns, which can cause problems in motor control, contribute to poor performance, and increase tension in the tissue. Quite often several different types of myofascial dysfunction overlap and may not be easy to decide which problems came first. In acute cases, treatment planning is easier because the altered area of myofascial tone or texture is still visible. In chronic cases, the therapist should focus on their palpation findings and try different treatment approaches (eg, relax tight and tensioned tissue, activate inactive areas, or improve range of movement). In many chronic cases, the most clinically significant findings are pain, joint stiffness, or lack of myofascial mobility. Affected horses may have concurrent behavioral issues such as fear, anger, or lack of trust. These horses often display signs of poor performance where they may have refusals in competitions or easily fatigue.

Suggestions for a myofascial treatment plan when a horse has more pain than stiffness or movement dysfunction:

- *Tier 1*—light touch techniques
- *Tier 2*—slow gliding techniques
- *Tier 3*—light mobilization and manipulation

Suggestions for a myofascial treatment plan when a horse has more stiffness and movement dysfunctions than pain:

- *Tier 1*—cross-fiber friction massage
- *Tier 2*—combinations of slower and faster techniques and firmer mobilization and manipulation
- *Tier 3*—ischemic compression

DISCUSSION

Myofascial treatment should aim to improve the performance and well-being of the horse. Proper treatment and rehabilitation programs include individualized exercises and incorporate a progressive plan of improving the body. Underlying pathologic condition can alter the body's capacity to heal, which needs to be closely monitored if the horse is not reacting the way you expect to the applied treatment. However, studies show that bony changes that are visible on radiographs are not necessarily causing pain or clinical signs that the horse is expressing.[24] It is always important to try to find the reason why the horse is not performing well, showing pain, or feeling unhappy by using different examination modalities from observation, palpation, manual testing, radiography, thermography, or scintigraphy to form a picture so that the different clinical pieces fit together.

If the treatment progression of the horse has stopped or if the horse is not improving as expected after treatment, check for any underlying pathologic condition and the effects of the saddle, bridle, bit, and the rider. Crooked and tense riders can induce myofascial tension within the horse's body. As sensitive animals, horses can easily mirror the myofascial problems of the rider. Also checking the overall management of the horse might be necessary (eg, shoeing, feeding, stable).

Treatment outcomes can be evaluated with observation of the static and dynamic posture, analyzing the movement quality and quantity, and by palpating the tissue texture and elasticity (**Fig. 9**). The rider and the owner should also monitor the clinical

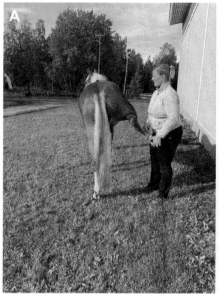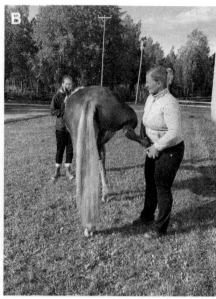

Fig. 9. Evaluation of passive joint motion is useful to evaluate the effectiveness of myofascial treatments. Pelvic limb abduction before (*A*) and after (*B*) myofascial treatment. (*Courtesy of* Johanna Kuuppo.)

signs and behavioral changes after treatment, so these can be also used as evaluation parameters to guide further treatment approaches. Our goal should be a happy horse, who is willing to perform with us according to the disciplines they are trained for.

CLINICS CARE POINTS

- Try to locate the source of the pain or dysfucntion with active and passive movement assessment and palpation.
- Vary myofascial treatment techniques according to the situation.
- Assess and re-assess treatment outcomes before and after treatment.
- Plan rehabilitation process and treatment protocol carefully.

DISCLOSURE

The author has nothing to disclose.

SUPPLEMENTARY DATA

Supplementary data related to this article can be found online at https://doi.org/10.1016/j.cveq.2022.06.007.

REFERENCES

1. Adstrum S, Hedley G, Schleip R, et al. Defining the fascial system. J Bodyw Mov Ther 2017;21:173–7.

2. Zügel M, Maganaris CN, Wilke J, et al. Consensus statement: Fascial tissue research in sports medicine: from molecules to tissue adaptation, injury and diagnostics. Br J Sports Med 2018. https://doi.org/10.1136/bjsports-2018-099308.

3. Fede C, Pirri C, Fan C, et al. A Closer Look at the Cellular and Molecular Components of the Deep/Muscular Fasciae. Int J Mol Sci 2021;22:1411.

4. Van Der Berg F. Extracellular Matrix. In: Schleip R, editor. Fascia – the tensional network of the human fascia. Churchill Livingstone Elsevier, England: Elsevier; 2012.

5. Ricard-Blum S. The collagen family. Cold Spring Harb Perspect Biol 2011;3(1): a004978.

6. Stecco C. Functional atlas of the human fascial system. Oxford, England: Churchill Livingstone, Elsevier; 2015.

7. Schleip R, Jäger H, Klingler W. What is 'fascia'? A review of different nomenclatures. J Bodyw Mov Ther 2012 Oct;16(4):496–502. https://doi.org/10.1016/j.jbmt. 2012.08.001. Epub 2012 Aug 22. PMID: 23036881.

8. Waqas A, Kulikowska M, Ahlmann T, et al. A comparative multi-site and whole-body assessment of fascia in the horse and dog: a detailed histological investigation. J Anat 2019;235(6):1065–77.

9. Luomala T, Mika P, Jouko H, et al. Case study: could ultrasound and elastography visualized densified areas inside the deep fascia? J Bodyw Mov Ther 2014;18(3): 462–8.

10. Menon RG, Oswald SF, Raghavan P, et al. $T_{1\rho}$-Mapping for Musculoskeletal Pain Diagnosis: Case Series of Variation of Water Bound Glycosaminoglycans Quantification before and after Fascial Manipulation® in Subjects with Elbow Pain. Int J Environ Res Public Health 2020;17(3):708.

11. Klingler W. Physiology and biochemistry in Fascia in sport and movement. Scotland, UK: Handspring; 2015.

12. Luomala T, Pihlman M. A practical guide to fascial manipulation – an evidence- and clinical based approach. Oxford, England: Elsevier; 2016.

13. Wakuri H. Cleavage Line Patterns of the Skin in the Horse. Okajimas Folia Anat Jpn 1990;67(5):351–63.

14. Schleip R, Findley T, Chaitow L, et al. Fascia. The tensional network of the human body. Oxford, England: Churchill & Livingstone, Elsevier; 2012.

15. Langevin HM. Fascia Mobility, Proprioception, and Myofascial Pain. Life 2021; 11(7):668.

16. Langevin H, Fox JR, Koptiuch C, et al. Reduced thoracolumbar fascia shear strain in human chronic low back pain. BMC Musculoskelet Disord 2011;12:203.

17. Stecco A, Meneghini A, Stern R, et al. Ultrasonography in myofascial neck pain: randomized clinical trial for diagnosis and follow-up. Surg Radiol Anat 2014;36: 243–53.

18. Schilder A, Hoheisel U, Magerl W, et al. Sensory findings after stimulation of the thoracolumbar fascia with hypertonic saline suggest its contribution to low back pain. Pain 2014;155(2):222–31.

19. Mense S. Innervation of the thoracolumbar fascia. 2019. Eur J Transl Myol 2019; 29(3):151–8.

20. Fede C, Albertin G, Petrelli L, et al. Hormone receptor expression in human fascial tissue. Eur J Histochem 2016;60(4):2710.

21. Walker S, Trotter P, Swaney W, et al. C-tactile afferents: Cutaneous mediators of oxytocin release during affiliative tactile interactions? 2017. Neuropeptides 2017;64:27–38.

22. Smith AV, Proops L, Grounds K, et al. Functionally relevant responses to human facial expressions of emotion in the domestic horse (Equus caballus). Biol Lett 2016;12:20150907.
23. Wathan J, Burrows A, Waller B, et al. EquiFACS: The equine facial action coding system. PLoS One 2015. https://doi.org/10.1371/journal.pone.0131738.
24. Zimmerman M, Dyson S, Murray R. Comparison of radiographic and scintigraphic findings of the spinous processes in the equine thoracolumbar region. J Vet Radiol Ultrasound 2011. https://doi.org/10.1111/j.1740-8261.2011.01845.x.

Spinal Mobilization and Manipulation in Horses

Kevin K. Haussler, DVM, DC, PhD[a],*, Tim N. Holt, DVM[b]

KEYWORDS

- Horse • Manual therapy • Chiropractic • Osteopathy • Physical therapy • Back pain
- Stiffness • Muscle hypertonicity

KEY POINTS

- Spinal mobilization and manipulation techniques provide important diagnostic and therapeutic approaches that are not otherwise available for addressing musculoskeletal pain, stiffness, and muscle hypertonicity in horses.
- Most musculoskeletal diagnostic procedures are used to localize a structural lesion; however, a more clinically relevant approach from a sports medicine and rehabilitation perspective is to focus on the functional status of the patient.
- Examination procedures include static and dynamic assessments of the quantity and the quality of both active and passive spinal movements.
- Clinical guidelines and tiered treatment approaches have not been developed but are much needed for the effective management of axial skeleton pain and dysfunction in horses.

 Video content accompanies this article at http://www.vetequine.theclinics.com

INTRODUCTION

Manual therapy is defined as the application of the hands to the body with a diagnostic or therapeutic intent . [1] There is a wide array of manual techniques used to treat axial skeleton pain, stiffness, and muscle hypertonicity. Of the different types of manual techniques that are used routinely in veterinary medicine, mobilization, or manipulation have the most evidence for producing beneficial clinical effects in horses.[2–5] Mobilization techniques use graded forces to displace musculoskeletal tissues and can generally be categorized into soft tissue or articular-based approaches.[6] Soft tissue mobilization typically focuses on restoring physiologic motion to the skin and

[a] Equine Orthopaedic Research Center, Department of Clinical Sciences, Colorado State University, 2350 Gillette Drive, 1621 Campus Delivery, Fort Collins, CO 80523-1621, USA;
[b] Integrated Livestock Management, Department of Clinical Sciences, Colorado State University, Veterinary Teaching Hospital, 300 West Drake Road, Fort Collins, CO, 80523, USA
* Corresponding author.
E-mail address: kevin.haussler@colostate.edu

Vet Clin Equine 38 (2022) 509–523
https://doi.org/10.1016/j.cveq.2022.06.008
0749-0739/22/© 2022 Elsevier Inc. All rights reserved.

underlying fascia, ligaments, and myotendinous structures with the aim of reducing pain, increasing tissue extensibility, and improving function. Joint mobilization is characterized as repetitive passive joint movements with the purpose of restoring normal articular motion.[7] Manipulation is characterized by the application of a non-repetitive, high-velocity, low-amplitude (HVLA) thrust directed at spinal or appendicular articulations.[8] Osteopathic techniques include a diverse array of diagnostic and treatment approaches that range from articular, myofascial, vascular, lymphatic, and neural techniques, which makes categorization of the type of applied therapy difficult.[9] In addition, it may not be clinically useful to categorize manual therapies into "stretching exercises" versus "mobilization" procedures as the descriptions are often poorly described and there may be a large overlap in the mechanism of action and clinical effects of the applied manual techniques.

Manual therapy implies using the hand to treat; however, instrument-assisted and electromechanical forms of manipulation have also been developed for use in humans to manage musculoskeletal disorders.[10] In horses, instrument-assisted manipulation (ie, activator) is reported to have a peak effect 7 days posttreatment.[11] Spinal mobilization and manipulation have reported maximal effects in horses after three treatment sessions at weekly intervals.[12] In humans, comparisons of the effectiveness of mobilization, instrument-assisted, and manual manipulation have been reported with no one type of therapy shown to be more effective than the others.[13,14] To date, there have not been any direct comparisons between the efficacy of manual versus instrument-assisted manipulation in horses.

Equine osteopathic evaluation and treatment procedures have been described in case reports, but no formal hypothesis-driven research exists.[15,16] Equine osteopathic studies often incorporate sedation or general anesthesia, but it is not clear if horses treated under sedation responded differently from horses treated under general anesthesia.[16–18] General statements provided by one author suggest that treating under general anesthesia produces more favorable results and was the preferred technique despite the inherent risks and added costs.[16] However, the authors also reported that general anesthesia was used for horses with intransigent or chronic issues, which would suggest that the prognosis for these cases might be worse than more subacute cases.

General categories of manual therapies based on varying tissue depths of application and the presence or absence of induced joint movement.

- Touch therapies
  - Gentle techniques that use a light hand contact or touch to affect superficial tissues and neurologic responses
  - Applied with the intent of interspecies bonding, calming, and retraining cutaneous sensations
- Myofascial techniques
  - Variety of techniques that use superficial to deep manual pressure or friction to mobilize skin, fascia, and muscles
  - Applied with the intent of increasing tissue compliance and reducing pain
- Stretching exercises
  - Active or passive movements that induce tension or lengthening of periarticular soft tissues and the associated articulations
  - Applied with the intent of increasing overall flexibility or joint range of motion
- Mobilization
  - Induced soft tissue displacement or graded amplitudes of joint movement
  - Applied with the intent of reducing pain and increasing tissue compliance or joint range of motion

- Manipulation
  - Characterized by HVLA thrusts applied to articulations or periarticular soft tissues
  - Applied with the intent of reducing pain, stiffness, and muscle hypertonicity

CLINICAL RELEVANCE

Detailed spinal evaluation procedures that incorporate mobilization techniques provide important diagnostic approaches for identifying and localizing axial skeleton problems in horses that are not otherwise available in veterinary medicine.[7] The sole reliance of diagnosing neck, back, or sacropelvic pain based on an owner's complaint and a precursory superficial palpation that precipitates an avoidance response is solely inadequate for most affected patients. In addition, the heavy reliance on diagnostic imaging to provide a structural or pathoanatomic diagnosis is often misguided, unless coupled with a through clinical history, static and dynamic observations, detailed soft tissue and osseous palpation, active and passive joint motion, and assessment of the quality and quantity of induced spinal reflexes. Pain, stiffness, and muscle hypertonicity are the principal clinical signs associated with axial skeleton issues and are all functional manifestations of underlying spinal inflammation or pathology.[19] Although the focus of most musculoskeletal diagnostic procedures is to localize a structural lesion, a more useful and clinically relevant approach from a sports medicine and rehabilitation perspective is to focus on the functional status and potential impairments of the equine patient.

Treatment effects can be generally categorized into disease-modifying and symptom-modifying. Although disease modification is the preferred or desired outcome, it is often difficult to achieve. As humans can describe sensations associated with their illness (ie, symptoms) and animals cannot, then reporting clinical signs are only possible in horses. Therefore, treatment effects are based on observed clinical signs, which may have a structural basis (eg, cross-sectional area, osteophyte, laceration), or more commonly a functional basis associated with reduced weight bearing, lack of impulsion, or weakness. As most structural lesions (eg, articular process osteoarthritis) are not amendable to a structural correction (eg, resection), then the primary treatment approach is to address the associated pain and dysfunction, which are largely amendable to functional treatment approaches and form the foundational basis for the identification of specific and actionable rehabilitation issues and the associated treatment plans. Therefore, the goal of spinal rehabilitation in horses with clinical signs of back pain or dysfunction is to influence the functional or clinical aspects by reducing the associated pain and epaxial muscle hypertonicity while also improving proprioception, flexibility, and core stability. From a surgical perspective, the only treatment option for horses with impinged spinous processes might be to address the osseous impingement observed on radiographs without full consideration of concurrent functional deficits. From the owner or patient perspective, there is often less concern about the structural aspects of the disease process and more focus is placed on resolution of the unremitting pain and loss of function.

Pathoanatomic diagnosis: It describes a structural or tissue-based pathology

- Diagnosis is based primarily on abnormal structural findings identified on physical examination, diagnostic imaging, and gross or histologic evaluation
  - Example: Radiologic diagnosis of impinged spinous processes
- Treatment goal is to physically remove the structural lesion
  - Example: Interspinous ligament desmotomy or spinous process resection

Functional diagnosis: It describes impairments in movement, activities of daily living, or athletic performance.

- Diagnosis is based on a through medical and performance history, observation, detailed spinal evaluation, and laboratory tests
  - Example: Severe epaxial muscle hypertonicity and trunk stiffness
- Treatment goal is to reduce pain and improve function
  - Example: Acupuncture and baited stretches

SPINAL EVALUATION PROCEDURES

A detailed manual evaluation of the axial skeleton includes a collection of diagnostic techniques that use the hands to evaluate and form an assessment of the structural and functional features of soft tissues, bony landmarks, articulations, and status of the neurologic system. Examination procedures include static and dynamic assessments of the quantity (eg, joint range of motion) and the quality of both active and passive movements.

A structured format for examining the axial skeleton includes (1) observation, (2) soft tissue palpation, (3), osseous palpation, (4) joint mobilization, (5) induced spinal reflexes, and (6) assessing active joint range of motion.

Static observation involves visual inspection of the stationary patient and includes assessing behavior, mental status, response to environmental distractions, conformation, posture, body condition score, hair coat quality, muscle development, and symmetry of topographic structures. Dynamic observation involves examination of a patient in motion or while performing a specific task. Functional assessments include response to environmental or external stimuli, owner or handler interactions, proprioception, coordination, balance, strength, active range of joint motion, gait evaluation, transitions, response to applied tack, the quality of motion under saddle, and response to the rider's cues.

Digital palpation includes a detailed examination and assessment of cutaneous responses (eg, acupoint reactivity) and structural and functional aspects of specific soft tissue layers and osseous landmarks. Palpation within the stationary patient includes assessing the nociceptive responses to touch and light pressure, and localizing changes in temperature, tone, texture, and tissue pliability. Soft tissue palpation includes assessing the quality and quantity of skin movement, fascial mobility, and muscle tone and development. The hair and skin are lightly palpated to identify changes in texture, skin nodules, and mobility. The skin is then gently mobilized using a flat hand contact to induce circular or orthogonal movements to evaluate the ease and mobility of the superficial fascia while monitoring for restricted motion, skin wrinkles, and any pain responses (Video 1). The superficial muscles are similarly assessed for tone and localized pain responses (Video 2). Deeper pressure is then applied to identify hypertonic bands or regions of muscle hypertonicity within deeper myofascial tissue layers. Common sites of myofascial pain and hypertonicity include the brachiocephalicus, triceps, spinalis, longissimus, and middle gluteal muscles. Allodynia is defined as a nociceptive response to normally non-noxious stimuli (eg, brushing, saddle placement) and is common in horses with clinical signs of myofascial or neuropathic pain. The thoracolumbar fascia is commonly affected in horses with back pain and can be systematically palpated from the withers to sacral region using firm digital pressure applied with the index finger and thumb lateral to the dorsal midline (Video 3).

Osseous palpation of the axial skeleton is limited due to the large overlying muscle mass and the deep location of most vertebral structures. Within the cervical region, the wing of the atlas (C1) is the most readily palpable osseous landmark. Although the transverse processes of the cervical vertebrae can be localized in most horses, the deeper articular processes are often difficult to palpate; however, joint function can be readily assessed with passive lateral bending (Video 4). Within the thoracolumbar region, the dorsal aspect of the spinous processes (Video 5) and the lateral rib cage are routinely assessed to identify localized pain responses. The tuber sacral and tuber coxae are readily palpated and serve as important attachment sites for sacropelvic ligaments and gluteal musculature.

Joint mobilization techniques are used to provide a much-needed assessment of the quantity and quality of passive vertebral segment motion. Passive joint range of motion should be evaluated from global and segmental perspectives. General screening techniques are used to assess the overall ease and ability of flexion–extension (Video 6) and lateral bending (Video 7) movements of the trunk and pelvis (Video 8). Spinal reflexes are used to assess the quality and quantity of active trunk motion by applying controlled noxious stimulation along (1) the ventral sternum to induce trunk elevation, (2) during simultaneous girth and contralateral croup region to induce overall trunk elevation and lateral bending, and (3) bilaterally at the sacrocaudal junction to induce pelvic flexion and caudal trunk elevation. Applying caudal tail traction can be used to evaluate lumbosacral pain and muscle activation. Active range of motion of the cervical and thoracolumbar regions is evaluated by using baited stretches to assess the quality and quantity of guided movements to predetermined landmarks. All passive and active joint motion techniques are used to localize and grade the severity of stiffness, pain responses, and musculoskeletal coordination.

CLINICAL INDICATIONS

Equine mobilization studies include osteopathic reports on the treatment of axial skeleton pain and stiffness (**Table 1**).[16–18] Significant medical histories often include behavioral or temperament changes, apprehension when saddled, and reduced ridden performance.[17] Static physical examination findings include the inability to stand squarely on all four limbs, epaxial muscle hypertonicity or atrophy, and signs of pelvic asymmetry. Subjective observation assesses changes in stride length, inconsistent limb placement, asymmetric pelvic motion, head and neck elevation combined with trunk lordosis, and the inability to back up in a straight line.[17]

Equine spinal manipulation studies primarily evaluate changes in thoracolumbar nociceptive thresholds (ie, back pain) and concurrent trunk stiffness and epaxial

Table 1
Summary of scientific literature evaluating the clinical effects of spinal mobilization and manipulation

Indication	Treatment Methods
Cervical	
Pain or stiffness	Osteopathy (with sedation, general anesthesia)[16–18]
Thoracolumbar	
Acute pain	Manipulation[20]
Chronic pain	Caudal tail traction[26] Manipulation[11,21,25]
Muscle hypertonicity	Manipulation[22]
Stiffness	Caudal trunk displacement[27] Osteopathy (with sedation, general anesthesia)[16,17] Manipulation[12,23,24]

muscle hypertonicity (Video 9).[11,12,20-25] Experimental studies of equine manipulation include HVLA thrusts applied bilaterally at standardized thoracolumbar locations in actively ridden horses participating in collegiate programs[12,21,22] or with experimentally induced spinous process pain.[23] In contrast, clinical studies typically address HVLA treatments at variable vertebral locations with localized signs of pain or joint stiffness within individual horses.[11,20,24,25]

CLINICAL EFFICACY

There is a wide variety of outcome parameters that have been used to evaluate the efficacy of spinal mobilization and manipulation techniques in horses.

Muscle Tone and Activity

Epaxial muscle tone, as measured by a mechanical tissue indenter, decreased significantly after a single HVLA treatment session by 13% compared with 0% change within control horses.[22] Similarly, muscle activity as measured by superficial electromyography showed a significant decrease of $21 \pm 7\%$ within the treatment group compared with $6 \pm 5\%$ in the control group. A single HVLA treatment session abolished myofascial sensitivity assessed with digital palpation and improved measures of muscle function using static bioimpedance and dynamic acoustic myography for up to 3 days posttreatment.[25]

Spinal Reflexes

In horses with acute back pain, significant improvements in the quality and amplitudes of spinal motion associated with induced thoracic (28%) and pelvic flexion (28%) reflexes were reported after spinal manipulation.[20] There were no significant treatment effects on the ability to resist caudal traction applied to the tail or the response to tuber sacral compression in this study.

Mechanical Nociceptive Thresholds

In a second study, caudal tail traction induced significant changes in mechanical nociceptive threshold (MNT) values across 10 lumbopelvic landmarks with an overall increase of 12 N/cm^2 (range 9 to 17 N/cm^2), which indicated heighted nociceptive thresholds (ie, less pain).[26] Within actively ridden horses without overt signs of back pain, MNT values were significantly increased by 27% after a single instrument-assisted HVLA treatment session 1 week posttreatment compared with < 1% change within both the active and inactive control groups.[11] In a separate study, spinal manipulation applied weekly for 3 weeks significantly increased MNT values within the treatment group by $11 \pm 7\%$, compared with the control group ($5 \pm 6\%$).[21] In a study that evaluated the effects of low-level laser therapy and spinal manipulation in horses with acute back pain, three spinal manipulation sessions produced a significant treatment group effect of 2% across pooled MNT values compared with no significant improvement (−4%) when manipulation was combined with low-level laser therapy.[20]

Thoracolumbar Flexibility

In horses with experimentally induced back pain, vertical trunk displacements increased 15% (range 7% to 25%) after HVLA compared with 0% (range −4% to 7%) in the control group.[23] In actively ridden horses without overt back pain, spinal flexibility as measured by passive vertical displacement of the trunk increased $16 \pm 7\%$ immediately after HVLA treatment across five thoracolumbar sites (T14–L6) compared with $0 \pm 3\%$ with mobilization alone.[12] However, vertical displacement measured 1 week after spinal manipulation or mobilization showed an increase in spinal flexibility of 10 ± 5% within the mobilization group compared with 5 ± 4% in the spinal manipulation group. These findings suggest an immediate effect on spinal flexibility due to HVLA treatment versus a delayed effect associated with spinal mobilization. After 3 weeks of once weekly HVLA treatment sessions, vertical displacement increased by 40% from baseline values compared with 19% with spinal mobilization alone.[12]

Motion Analysis

Induced caudal weight shifting caused significant flattening (ie, reduced lordosis) of the dorsal trunk contour as measured from T10 to L3 with overall changes in vertical displacement of 11 mm (range 1 to 20 mm) and thoracolumbar angles of 3.4° (range 0.2° to 7.2°).[27] In a separate study that evaluated ridden horses with back pain, a single session of spinal manipulation had minor, variable effects on vertebral and pelvic kinematics as measured at the walk and trot.[24] Thoracolumbar and pelvic range of motion tended to increase directly after treatment but decreased 3 weeks later compared with baseline values. Specific changes included increased thoracolumbar sagittal motion and symmetry of pelvic rotation. No significant changes were noted in stride parameters or cervical vertebral motion patterns.[24]

Visual Analog Scales

In horses with acute back pain, a veterinarian-derived visual analog scale (VAS) of back pain severity and spinal function showed no treatment effect over three spinal manipulation sessions compared with a significant improvement in these parameters within a low-level laser therapy group.[20] Owner reported VAS scores decreased (ie, reduced back pain) across sessions; however, the changes were not significant within spinal manipulation or combined manipulation and laser therapy groups.

Owner Surveys of Performance

The treatment of equine neck pain and stiffness using mobilization techniques under anesthesia produced clinical improvement based exclusively on owner reports as early as 2 days, with 95% of horses improved within 2 weeks posttreatment.[18] Based on owner reports, 95% of horses were reported to be improved at least 6 months posttreatment using osteopathic techniques with complete resolution in 74% and partial improvement in 26% of patients.[16] In another equine osteopathic study using owner surveys, return to work was reported at 6 to 12 weeks in 90% of horses, which had all undergone prior unsuccessful conventional treatment.[17] A long-term follow-up (>12 months) based on rider assessments showed 53% of horses continued in normal work, 31% worked at a lower level, and 16% were unrideable. These investigators suggested that the success of osteopathic treatment depends on the owner's ability to return horses slowly to work, reestablished patterns of normal tissue function with therapeutic exercises or rehabilitation, and repeat treatment sessions using manual therapies.[17]

Lameness Evaluation

No significant changes in objective measures of limb lameness have been reported in actively ridden horses treated with spinal manipulation.[25]

CLINICAL GUIDELINES

Evidence-based clinical guidelines for the management of neck and back pain are common in human medicine and have been developed to better assess the clinical efficacy and cost-effectiveness of patient-based care versus the usual standard of care or a "one-size-fits-all" primary care strategy.[28] The guidelines are typically based on categorization of the patient's clinical signs (eg, acute vs chronic, microtrauma vs macrotrauma) and diagnostic testing (eg, presence of neurologic deficits, specific pathoanatomic diagnosis) into specific three clinical subgroups (ie, nonspecific pain, neurologic deficits, or specific pathology).[28] Treatment recommendations are then provided based on systematic reviews of randomized controlled clinical trials with an overall ranking of treatments based on low, moderate, and high levels of therapeutic efficacy. In human patients with acute back pain, most guidelines recommend avoiding bed rest and low levels of activity.[29] For chronic back pain patients, a multidisciplinary approach is typically recommended, which includes exercise, rehabilitation, and spinal mobilization or manipulation.[30,31]

Unfortunately, similar guidelines have not been developed for the management of axial skeleton pain and dysfunction in horses, due mostly to the lack of a sufficient number of controlled clinical trials.[32] Data from the current equine mobilization and manipulation studies suggest that clinical effects are often noted after a single treatment session.[11,22,24–26] Most spinal manipulation studies assess changes in outcome parameters immediately posttreatment; however, short-term effects have been reported at 2 to 6 days[25] and up to 1 to 3 weeks after a single HVLA treatment session.[11,24] The effects of a single treatment session are not likely useful in formulating practice guidelines where several treatment sessions may be required to achieve the desired therapeutic effects.[24] Recurrent treatment sessions for spinal manipulation have included three treatment sessions over 3 to 5 days[20] or treatment once weekly for 3 weeks.[12,21] Osteopathic treatment under sedation has been applied every 2 to 6 weeks for an average of six treatment sessions.[17] Owing to the wide diversity in applied treatments, variable treatment sites, and the total number of applied mobilizations or HVLA thrusts per treatment session, it is difficult to synthesize the available information into clinically useful dosage recommendations at this time.

In humans, tiered treatment guidelines have been developed based on the patient's needs and the severity or complexity of clinical signs.[33,34] Most tiered treatment recommendations are based on pain type and severity; however, measures of overall function are also considered.[35] Tier 1 treatment plans are designed for managing acute back pain episodes. Tier 2 treatment recommendations focus on more severe or recurrent back pain. Tier 3 treatment is geared toward unrelenting back pain that requires surgical intervention or provides palliative care for patients with end-stage disease. Again, similar tiered treatment guidelines do not currently exist in equine practice but are much needed to help guide practitioners in the treatment of axial skeleton pain and dysfunction.

The proposed tiered treatment options for horses with chronic back pain and stiffness.

Tier 1
- Baited stretches[36]
- Acupuncture[37]
- Low-level laser therapy[20]
- Spinal mobilization and manipulation[12]

Tier 2
- Diagnostic imaging
- Extracorporeal shockwave therapy[38]
- Intra-articular or periarticular joint injections[39]
  - Articular process joints

- ○ Intertransverse joints
Tier 3
- Surgical consultation
  - ○ Interspinous ligament desmotomy[40]
  - ○ Spinous process resection[41]
- Epidural corticosteroids[42]

CLINICAL CASE

A 6-year-old Quarter Horse gelding was referred for loss of performance due to a suspected painful back. The horse was used in competitive barrel racing and over the past month has had slower race times and the turns around the barrels have become wider and less controlled. The horse has lost his home speed and even hesitates to start the run. The owner has noted that the horse no longer likes to be brushed and resists saddle placement. Once the saddle is on, the horse is fine, but does not seem to be happy. The referring veterinarian has examined the horse and is suspicious of low to mid-grade back pain as the horse does not allow palpation of any type over the entire dorsal trunk with the most intense pain response and the area of concern located from T8 to the lumbosacral junction. The referring veterinarian medicated the horse with phenylbutazone with little effect and has now referred the horse for further diagnostics and integrative therapies.

Tier 1 Examination and Treatment

On routine physical examination, there were no significant findings. A full-body myofascial examination (ie, head, neck, trunk, limbs) was completed to identify restricted myofascial movement and localize reactive sites within the cutaneous (eg, acupuncture) or muscular (eg, trigger points) tissues. The findings from the myofascial examination confirm the presence of allodynia localized to the area from T8 to the lumbosacral junction. An evaluation of passive joint range of motion of the thoracolumbar region confirmed generalized joint stiffness and abnormal pain responses. The tier 1 treatment plan for addressing the epaxial muscle pain and stiffness consisted of the following:

- Low-level laser therapy focused on the most painful regions of the dorsal trunk[20]
- Passive spinal mobilization in flexion, extension, and lateral bending to induce trunk motion[23]
- Induced lateral bending of the trunk by applying pressure to the lateral rib cage with the cranial hand while pulling laterally with the caudal hand on the tail to induce rhythmic rib cage and trunk mobilization
- Active joint range of motion using baited stretches directed toward the tarsal region while stabilizing the pelvis with static lateral tail traction to induce trunk flexion and lateral bending[43]
- Light tissue vibration with a hand-held massage unit over all sensitive dorsal trunk areas and large muscle groups to stimulate muscle relaxation
- Light tissue massage progressing to deeper tissue and trigger point therapy, as tolerated to reduce myofascial pain and hypertonicity[44,45]
- Walking backwards for 20 feet at a slow speed and in straight lines over level ground to retrain motor control and coordination of the dorsal and ventral muscle chains of the trunk
- Ice massage to residual painful regions by applying ice in small continuous circles for 10 minutes

- Recommend discontinuing all ridden exercise with monitored turnout in a small field to allow grazing and stretching of the dorsal trunk soft tissues
- Discuss with the owner the feasibility of doing at-home exercises at least 3 times per week, which would include active hand walking, ice massage, gentle manual massage, lateral rib cage mobilization, and baited stretches
- Repeat myofascial and spinal evaluation in 7 to 14 days

Tier 2 Examination and Treatment

The owner reported a good response to treatment, but the horse is still not perceived to be normal. The entire myofascial and spinal evaluation were repeated with increasing depth and intensity of soft tissue palpation and amplitude of passive joint mobilization.. The horse allowed a more in-depth evaluation of the articulations of the rib cage, caudal lumbar vertebrae, and lumbosacral and sacroiliac joints via rhythmic passive joint mobilization. The tier 2 treatment plan for addressing the residual epaxial muscle pain and trunk stiffness consisted of the following options:

- Repeat application of low-level laser therapy, passive trunk mobilization, and active range of motion with baited stretches to reduce thoracolumbar pain and stiffness
- Apply acupuncture and add electroacupuncture as tolerated to the epaxial musculature of the trunk to reduce pain[37]
- Apply HVLA thrusts (spinal manipulation) to areas of pain, stiffness, and muscle hypertonicity[12]
- Apply topical nonsteroidal (diclofenac) to localized painful areas along the dorsal trunk
- Consider applying focused extracorporeal shockwave therapy over the most painful sites of the epaxial musculature using an 80-mm trode and over osseous landmarks using a 30-mm trode[38]
- Prescribe gabapentin for the chronic pain and methocarbamol for residual epaxial muscle hypertonicity for 30 days
- Increase exercise intensity and duration with walk, canter transitions in a round pen or on a large circle with the lunge
- Add long-line work to help reestablish response to cues, coordination, and motor control
- Continue all prior at-home exercise recommendations
- Schedule next acupuncture session for 7 to 10 days and a second extracorporeal shockwave treatment, as indicated

Tier 3 Examination and Treatment

The owner reported a good overall improvement, but the horse still seems to have some lingering pain and lack of desire to work. Recheck evaluation is 20 days since the last complete spinal examination. The tier 3 diagnostic and treatment plan consisted of the following options:

Advanced diagnostics
- Comprehensive limb lameness and neurologic examinations
- Isolate areas of clinical concern based on residual pain and stiffness within the thoracolumbar region
- Recommend percutaneous ultrasonographic examination of the supraspinous ligament, thoracolumbar fascia, dorsal sacroiliac ligaments, and caudal thoracic and lumbar articular processes[46]

- Recommend transrectal ultrasound to evaluate the ventral aspects of the lumbo-sacral, intertransverse, and sacroiliac joints[47]
- Recommend radiographic imaging of the thoracolumbar spinous processes to evaluate for the presence of impinged spinous process and articular process joint osteoarthritis[48]
- Consider nuclear scintigraphy to identify focal increased radiopharmaceutical uptake[49]
- Consider diagnostic local anesthesia of the dorsal trunk or sacroiliac structures based on the radiographic, ultrasound, and nuclear scintigraphy findings[50,51]
- Expand the area of investigation to the head, neck, and pelvic regions
- Consider a complete blood count and serum biochemistry for evaluation of overall metabolic status and muscle enzyme levels

Treatment considerations

- Increase the intensity and frequency of acupuncture treatments to once or twice weekly
- Add Chinese herbal therapy[37]
- Complete the third extracorporeal shockwave treatment
- Recommend prescribed use of gabapentin and methocarbamol for another 30 days
- Consider periarticular or intra-articular corticosteroid injections of the affected thoracolumbar articular process[52]
- Consider incorporating mesotherapy of the trunk epaxial musculature to help reduce residual pain
- Depending on the diagnostic imaging findings, may consider a surgical consultation for treatment of impinged spinous processes[40,53]
- May consider treatment with epidural corticosteroids[54]
- Weekly rechecks for the next 3 weeks for repeated treatment with low-level laser therapy, acupuncture, myofascial work, joint mobilization, and spinal manipulation

Follow-up examinations and treatment resolved the horse's back pain and stiffness with a return to successful competition. This horse was effectively managed with conservative treatment options and remained in athletic competition with periodic manual therapy and acupuncture treatment, combined with at home exercises of massage and baited stretches. No diagnostic imaging or surgical procedures were required.

SUMMARY

The clinical indications for spinal mobilization and manipulation include pain, stiffness, muscle hypertonicity, lameness, and poor performance. Future studies need to establish quantitative and qualitative methods to specifically evaluate the effects of mobilization and manipulation, incorporate adequate control groups, provide long-term follow-up, and include evaluation of appendicular articulations.[32] Optimal technique indications and dosages also need to be help establish clinical guidelines and tiered treatment recommends for horses with axial skeleton pain and dysfunction.

CLINICS CARE POINTS

- An effective treatment plan is only as good as the diagnosis

- Spinal mobilization and manipulation have the highest level of evidence-based support as conservative treatment modalities for thoracolumbar pain and dysfunction in horses

DISCLOSURE

The authors have nothing to disclose.

SUPPLEMENTARY DATA

Supplementary data related to this article can be found online at https://doi.org/10.1016/j.cveq.2022.06.008.

REFERENCES

1. Haussler KK. Equine manual therapies in sport horse practice. Vet Clin North Am Equine Pract 2018;34(2):375–89.
2. Bergenstrahle A, Nielsen BD. Attitude and behavior of veterinarians surrounding the use of complementary and alternative veterinary medicine in the treatment of equine musculoskeletal pain. J Equine Vet Sci 2016;45:87–97.
3. Lange CD, Axiak Flammer S, Gerber V, et al. Complementary and alternative medicine for the management of orthopaedic problems in Swiss Warmblood horses. Vet Med Sci 2017;3(3):125–33.
4. Thirkell J, Hyland R. A survey examining attitudes towards equine complementary therapies for the treatment of musculoskeletal injuries. J Equine Vet Sci 2017;59:82–7.
5. Wilson JM, McKenzie E, Duesterdieck-Zellmer K. International survey regarding the use of rehabilitation modalities in horses. Front Vet Sci 2018;5:120.
6. Hesbach AL. Manual therapy in veterinary rehabilitation. Top Companion Anim Med. Mar 2014;29(1):20–3.
7. Haussler KK. Joint mobilization and manipulation for the equine athlete. Vet Clin North Am Equine Pract 2016;32(1):87–101.
8. Haussler KK. Review of manual therapy techniques in equine practice. J Equine Vet Sci 2009;29(12):849–69.
9. Licciardone JC. Osteopathic research: elephants, enigmas, and evidence. Osteopath Med Prim Care 2007;1:7.
10. Colloca CJ, Keller TS, Black P, et al. Comparison of mechanical force of manually assisted chiropractic adjusting instruments. J Manipulative Physiol Ther 2005;28(6):414–22.
11. Sullivan KA, Hill AE, Haussler KK. The effects of chiropractic, massage and phenylbutazone on spinal mechanical nociceptive thresholds in horses without clinical signs. Equine Vet J 2008;40(1):14–20.
12. Haussler KK, Martin CE, Hill AE. Efficacy of spinal manipulation and mobilisation on trunk flexibility and stiffness in horses: a randomised clinical trial. Equine Vet J Suppl 2010;38:695–702.
13. Gemmell H, Miller P. Comparative effectiveness of manipulation, mobilisation and the activator instrument in treatment of non-specific neck pain: a systematic review. Chiropr Osteopat 2006;14:7.
14. Shearar KA, Colloca CJ, White HL. A randomized clinical trial of manual versus mechanical force manipulation in the treatment of sacroiliac joint syndrome. J Manipulative Physiol Ther 2005;28(7):493–501.

15. Verschooten F. Osteopathy in locomotion problems of the horse: a critical evaluation. Vlaams Diergeneeskd Tijdschr 1992;61:116–20.

16. Pusey A, Colles C, Brooks J. Osteopathic treatment of horses - a retrospective study. Br Osteopathic J 1995;16:30–2.

17. Colles CM, Nevin A, Brooks J. The osteopathic treatment of somatic dysfunction causing gait abnormality in 51 horses. Equine Vet Educ 2014;26(3):148–55.

18. Ahern TJ. Cervical vertebral mobilization under anesthetic (CVMUA): A physical therapy for the treatment of cervico-spinal pain and stiffness. J Equine Vet Sci 1994;14(10):540–5.

19. Mayaki AM, Razak ISA, Adzahan NM, et al. Clinical assessment and grading of back pain in horses. Article. J Vet Sci 2020;21(6):10. e82.

20. Haussler KK, Manchon PT, Donnell JR, et al. Effects of low-level laser therapy and chiropractic care on back pain in Quarter Horses. J Equine Vet Sci 2020;86: 102891.

21. Haussler KK, Erb HN. Pressure algometry: objective assessment of back pain and effects of chiropractic treatment. Proc Amer Assoc Equine Pract 2003;49: 66–70.

22. Wakeling JM, Barnett K, Price S, et al. Effects of manipulative therapy on the longissimus dorsi in the equine back. Equine Comp Exerc Physiol 2006;3(3):153–60.

23. Haussler KK, Hill AE, Puttlitz CM, et al. Effects of vertebral mobilization and manipulation on kinematics of the thoracolumbar region. Am J Vet Res 2007; 68(5):508–16.

24. Gomez Alvarez CB, L'Ami JJ, Moffat D, et al. Effect of chiropractic manipulations on the kinematics of back and limbs in horses with clinically diagnosed back problems. Equine Vet J 2008;40(2):153–9.

25. Acutt EV, le Jeune SS, Pypendop BH. Evaluation of the effects of chiropractic on static and dynamic muscle variables in sport horses. J Equine Vet Sci 2019;73: 84–90.

26. Long K, McGowan CM, Hyytiäinen HK. Effect of caudal traction on mechanical nociceptive thresholds of epaxial and pelvic musculature on a group of horses with signs of back pain. J Equine Vet Sci 2020;93:103197.

27. Taylor F, Tabor G, Williams JM. Altered thoracolumbar position during application of craniocaudal spinal mobilisation in clinically sound leisure horses. Comp Exerc Physiol 2019;15(1):49–53.

28. Oliveira CB, Maher CG, Pinto RZ, et al. Clinical practice guidelines for the management of non-specific low back pain in primary care: an updated overview. Eur Spine J 2018;27(11):2791–803.

29. van Tulder M, Becker A, Bekkering T, et al. Chapter 3. European guidelines for the management of acute nonspecific low back pain in primary care. Eur Spine J 2006;15(Suppl 2):S169–91.

30. Chou R, Deyo R, Friedly J, et al. Nonpharmacologic therapies for low back pain: a systematic review for an american college of physicians clinical practice guideline. Ann Intern Med 2017;166(7):493–505.

31. Bussières AE, Stewart G, Al-Zoubi F, et al. Spinal manipulative therapy and other conservative treatments for low back pain: a guideline from the Canadian Chiropractic Guideline Initiative. J Manipulative Physiol Ther 2018;41(4):265–93.

32. Haussler KK, Hesbach AL, Romano L, et al. A systematic review of musculoskeletal mobilization and manipulation techniques used in veterinary medicine. Animals 2021;11(10):2787.

33. Palylyk-Colwell E, Wright MD. CADTH rapid response reports. Tiered care for chronic non-malignant pain: a review of clinical effectiveness, cost-effectiveness,

and guidelines. Ottawa: Canadian Agency for Drugs and Technologies in Health; 2019.

34. Smith EML, Bakitas MA, Homel P, et al. Preliminary assessment of a neuropathic pain treatment and referral algorithm for patients with cancer. J Pain Symptom Manage 2011;42(6):822–38.

35. Ellis BM, Conaghan PG. Reducing arthritis pain through physical activity: a new public health, tiered approach. Br J Gen Pract Oct 2017;67(663):438–9.

36. de Oliveira K, Soutello RVG, da Fonseca R, et al. Gymnastic training and dynamic mobilization exercises improve stride quality and increase epaxial muscle size in therapy horses. J Equine Vet Sci 2015;35(11):888–93.

37. Shmalberg J, Xie H, Memon MA. Horses referred to a teaching hospital exclusively for acupuncture and herbs: A three-year retrospective analysis. J Acupunct Meridian Stud 2019;12(5):145–50.

38. Trager LR, Funk RA, Clapp KS, et al. Extracorporeal shockwave therapy raises mechanical nociceptive threshold in horses with thoracolumbar pain. Equine Vet J 2020;52(2):250–7.

39. Birmingham SSW, Reed SM, Mattoon JS, et al. Qualitative assessment of corticosteroid cervical articular facet injection in symptomatic horses. Equine Vet Educ 2010;22(2):77–82.

40. Prisk AJ, Garcia-Lopez JM. Long-term prognosis for return to athletic function after interspinous ligament desmotomy for treatment of impinging and overriding dorsal spinous processes in horses: 71 cases (2012-2017). Article. Vet Surg 2019;48(7):1278–86.

41. Jacklin BD, Minshall GJ, Wright IM. A new technique for subtotal (cranial wedge) ostectomy in the treatment of impinging/overriding spinous processes: description of technique and outcome of 25 cases. Equine Vet J 2014;46(3):339–44.

42. Michielsen A, Schauvliege S. Epidural anesthesia and analgesia in horses. Vlaams Diergeneeskd Tijdschr 2019;88(4):233–40.

43. Clayton HM, Kaiser LJ, Lavagnino M, et al. Evaluation of intersegmental vertebral motion during performance of dynamic mobilization exercises in cervical lateral bending in horses. Am J Vet Res 2012;73(8):1153–9.

44. Kowalik S, Janczarek I, Kędzierski W, et al. The effect of relaxing massage on heart rate and heart rate variability in purebred Arabian racehorses. Ani Sci J 2017;88(4):669–77.

45. Kędzierski W, Janczarek I, Stachurska A, et al. Comparison of effects of different relaxing massage frequencies and different music hours on reducing stress level in race horses. J Equine Vet Sci 2017;53:100–7.

46. Fuglbjerg V, Nielsen JV, Thomsen PD, et al. Accuracy of ultrasound-guided injections of thoracolumbar articular process joints in horses: a cadaveric study. Equine Vet J 2010;42(1):18–22.

47. Boado A, Nagy A, Dyson S. Ultrasonographic features associated with the lumbosacral or lumbar 5-6 symphyses in 64 horses with lumbosacral-sacroiliac joint region pain (2012-2018). Equine Vet Educ 2020;32:136–43.

48. Cousty M, Retureau C, Tricaud C, et al. Location of radiological lesions of the thoracolumbar column in French trotters with and without signs of back pain. Vet Rec 2010;166(2):41–5.

49. van Zadelhoff C, Ehrle A, Merle R, et al. Thoracic processi spinosi findings agree among subjective, semiquantitative, and modified semiquantitative scintigraphic image evaluation methods and partially agree with clinical findings in horses with and without thoracolumbar pain. Vet Radiol Ultrasound 2019;60(2):210–8.

50. Derham AM, Schumacher J, O' Leary JM, et al. Implications of the neuroanatomy of the equine thoracolumbar vertebral column with regional anaesthesia and complications following desmotomy of the interspinous ligament. Equine Vet J 2021;53(4):649–55.

51. Delgado OBD, Louro LF, Rocchigiani G, et al. Ultrasound-guided erector spinae plane block in horses: a cadaver study. Vet Anaesth Analg 2021;48(4):577–84.

52. Cousty M, Firidolfi C, Geffroy O, et al. Comparison of medial and lateral ultrasound-guided approaches for periarticular injection of the thoracolumbar intervertebral facet joints in horses. Vet Surg 2011;40(4):494–9.

53. Derham AM, O'Leary JM, Connolly SE, et al. Performance comparison of 159 Thoroughbred racehorses and matched cohorts before and after desmotomy of the interspinous ligament. Vet J 2019;249:16–23.

54. van Loon JP, Menke ES, Doornenbal A, et al. Antinociceptive effects of low dose lumbosacral epidural ropivacaine in healthy ponies. Vet J 2012;193(1):240–5.

Clinical Application of Acupuncture in Equine Practice

Jennifer Repac, DVM. Diplomat ACVSMR[a],*, Emily Mangan, DVM[b],
Huisheng Xie, DVM, MS, PhD[c]

KEYWORDS

- Equine • Horse • Acupuncture • Chinese medicine • TCVM

KEY POINTS

- Acupuncture has been used to treat equine diseases in China for more than 2000 years.
- The use of acupuncture in equine practice has increased during the past few decades in the United States and other countries.
- A growing number of evidence-based studies have demonstrated the efficacy of this ancient medical modality.

INTRODUCTION

Traditional Chinese Veterinary Medicine (TCVM) has been used to treat disease and relieve pain in horses for more than 2000 years.[1,2] There are 4 main branches of TCVM: acupuncture, Chinese herbology, tui-na, and food therapy. Acupuncture is one of the most popular and commonly used complementary treatments in veterinary medicine due to its long history of use, increasing scientific evidence supporting efficacy, and inclusion in curriculum of United States veterinary colleges.[3–6] Acupuncture involves the stimulation of specific anatomic locations (acupoints) to create local and systemic responses in the body. It is a minimally invasive, practical, and inexpensive modality that can be used to treat several medical conditions. A recent study documenting cases at a teaching hospital reported that most of equine acupuncture referrals are for musculoskeletal conditions, followed by gastrointestinal disease and anhidrosis.[3] The most commonly used acupuncture methods include dry needle therapy, electroacupuncture, aquapuncture (point injection of vitamin B12 or pharmaceuticals), blood draw (hemoacupuncture), laser, acupressure, and moxibustion. In the past several decades, a growing body of research has demonstrated the

[a] University of Florida, College of Veterinary Medicine, 2015 Southwest 16th Avenue, Gainesville, FL 32608, USA; [b] Wisewood Integrative Veterinary Medicine, LLC, PO Box 608, Pleasant Hill, OR 97455, USA; [c] Chi University, 9650 West Highway 318, Reddick, FL 32686, USA
* Corresponding author.
E-mail address: jrepac@ufl.edu

Vet Clin Equine 38 (2022) 525–539
https://doi.org/10.1016/j.cveq.2022.07.001
0749-0739/22/© 2022 Elsevier Inc. All rights reserved.

neurochemical and endocrinological effects of acupuncture. Recent literature has demonstrated efficacy of acupuncture in horses for the treatment of back pain,[7-9] anxiety,[10] laminitis,[11-13] lameness,[2,14] sarcoidosis,[15] laryngeal hemiplegia,[16] and improving metabolic capacity in athletes.[17]

Mechanism of Action of Acupuncture

Acupuncture has neurophysiological effects in the body locally, at the level of the spinal cord, and at the brain. This is the reason why treatment of conditions often includes points located near as well as distant to the targeted area.[18-21]

Local effects:
- Inflammatory response leading to the release of leukotrienes, prostaglandins, bradykinin, and platelet activating factor
- Sympathetic release of β-endorphins and enkephalins
- Decrease in proinflammatory cytokines tumor necrosis factor (TNF)α,[22] interleukin (IL)-1β, and IL-6
- Decrease in nerve growth factor
- Release of mast cells leading to increase in adenosine triphoshate (ATP)[23] and vasodilation via release of histamine, heparin, and kinin protease
- Upregulate of cannabinoid (CB2) receptors
- Upregulate transient receptor potential vanilloid type-1) receptors[24]
- Stimulation of Aδ and C nociceptive nerve fibers
- Stimulation of nonnociceptive Aβ and Aα nerve fibers

Spinal cord mechanisms:
- Suppress N-methyl-D-aspartate via opioids, noradrenalin, and serotonin of dorsal horn neurons
- Decrease glial cell production, lowering release of TNFα, IL-1, IL-1β, COX-2, PGE2, and IL-6
- Increase the release of inhibitory γ-amino-butyric acid (GABA)
- Decrease in substance P

Brain mechanisms:
- Activate multiple areas of the brain (prefrontal cerebral cortex, medulla, periaquaductal gray, hypothalamus, midbrain, and pons)
- Release of enkephalins, noradrenaline, dopamine, serotonin, and β-endorphins lead to suppression of pain signals to the dorsal horn
- Release of oxytocin and ACTH release from the pituitary gland contribute to antinociception

Anatomy of Acupoints

In Chinese, acupoints are called *Shu-Xue*. *Shu* (腧) means transporting, distributing, or communication; *Xue* (穴) refers to a hole, outlet, or depression. Metaphorically, acupoints are hubs where internal energy gathers on the body surface. As the Chinese name suggests, acupoints are often externally palpable depressions. These loci were originally selected by ancient Traditional Chinese Medicine practitioners based on therapeutic effects triggered by stimulation.[6] However, scientific research has shown that many acupoints possess unique anatomic and histologic qualities.[18,24-28] These include local concentrations or sites of transmission:

- Lymphatics
- Nerve bundles
- Sympathetic chain (specific to the Bladder meridian)
- Capillaries and venules

- Fascial planes
- Motor points (where nerves penetrate muscle and tendon)
- Muscular junctions
- Common locations of myofascial trigger points
- Higher density of intercellular gap junctions leading to increased flow of nitric oxide (NO) and decreased electrical impedance

The original acupoints established in humans were translated into "transpositional points" appropriate for animal anatomy. There is also a collection of points created specifically for animals termed "classical points."[29]

Diagnostic quality of acupoints
The activation of parts of the brain by stimulation of distal acupoints has been demonstrated through studies using PET scans.[30]

Meridians

Most acupoints are grouped into 14 meridians (or "Regular" channels).[29] Each meridian follows a route from one end of the body to the other, like a road map. Twelve of these meridians are named after organs (eg, Kidney, Gallbladder, and Liver). The remaining 2 channels are the Governing Vessel and Conception Vessel meridians, which are located along the dorsal and ventral midline of the body, respectively. Each acupoint is named according to the meridian to which it belongs, followed by a number indicating its location in sequence. For instance, the first point on the Spleen meridian is named "SP-1."

Anatomically, meridians have been found to follow the course of peripheral nerves[31] and fascial planes.[32] The truncal points of the Bladder meridian affect visceral organs due to the sympathetic innervation of their respective myotomes.[33] Within the head, fascial acupoints tend to follow the course of the facial and trigeminal nerves from foramina to terminus.

Treatment Principles of Acupuncture

Pattern diagnosis
The central concept of TCVM is that the body is a complex interplay of flow of energies among systems.[34] Each of these components must be in balance in order to maintain the health of an organism. This parallels the hormonal and neurologic signaling in the Western medicine concept of biological homeostasis. TCVM therapy aims to rebalance these forces, using the body's innate ability to self-heal. A TCVM diagnosis is made through a combination of presenting complaint, patient history details (eg, sleep/wake cycles, urination patterns), signalment (eg, age, sex), and physical examination findings (eg, tongue color, pulse quality). A patient's personality, also known as constitution, may also support a particular diagnosis. As a result, a single Western diagnosis can present with variable TCVM diagnoses based on the pattern of TCVM clinical signs.

Acupuncture techniques

- *Dry needle:* This is the most commonly used form of acupuncture. Acupuncture needles are single-use and sterile, ranging from 20 to 32 gauge and 0.5 to 3.5 inches in length. Needle length is selected based on the depth of the targeted acupoint. Hypodermic needles (50–70 mm, 20–22 gauge) may also be used in cattle and horses.[20]
- *Electroacupuncture:* Electrical leads are connected to acupuncture needles, which are connected to a machine that generates electrical current. Compared

with dry needling, this provides a more long lasting and potent effect.[13] This particularly technique has been shown to activate Aβ and Aδ nerve fibers. The frequency of treatment has been shown to determine the neurochemical mediators released:[18]

- o *Low frequency* (2–10 Hz): Enkephalins, endorphins, noradrenergic, muscarinic, cholinergic
- o *Moderate high frequency* (50–100 Hz): Dynorphin, muscarinic, GABAergic
- o *High frequency* (200 Hz): Serotonin
- *Aquapuncture*: A variety of substances including pharmaceuticals, autologous blood, and commonly vitamin B12 (cobalamin) are injected into an acupoint using a sterile needle and syringe. This causes a localized distension of the area, thereby creating a longer lasting effect than a dry needle alone. Lower effective doses of injected medications (also called pharmacopuncture) can be achieved as reported in several veterinary studies.[35–37]
- *Hemoacupuncture:* A needle is briefly placed in an acupoint to induce a small amount of hemorrhage. This technique is most indicated for inflammatory conditions, such as laminitis.[11]
- *Moxibustion:* The lit end of a cigar-shaped roll of herbs (most commonly *Artemisia sinensis*, "mugwort") is held above the acupoint or a placed needle and is used to apply local heating. Sometimes, a slice of ginger is laid on the patient for thermal protection.

Acupoint selection

Once a TCVM diagnosis is obtained, acupoints are selected based on the goals of treatment. The most common basic methods of point selection are listed.[29]

- *Local point selection*: This includes selection of points located near the area of pathologic condition. For example, points located around the stifle can be used to treat stifle pain. A technique called "surround the dragon" in which needles are placed circumscribing a wound is another form of local point selection.
- *Meridian point selection*: If there is a specific organ of pathologic condition, points can be selected if they belong to that organ's meridian. For example, one may choose points along the Liver meridian to treat liver diseases.
- *Eight principles selection*: This method of point selection aims to rebalance TCVM concepts such as *Yin* versus *Yang* and hot versus cold.
- *Five Element point selection*: The 5 elements of TCVM (earth, fire, water, metal, and wood) each govern a set of organs and qualities. Points may be selected based on the interrelationship of these elements.
- *Acupuncture point scan*: A scanning examination is performed by applying light touch along the horse's body to reveal areas of hypersensitivity known as "*A-shi*" points. This process has been shown to have an 82% sensitivity and 78% specificity in detecting forelimb and hindlimb lameness.[38] Acupoints can be selected in these areas to target myofascial trigger points.

Duration and frequency of acupuncture sessions

The suggested duration of acupuncture treatment in horses typically ranges from 15 to 30 minutes per session, with 1 session per 1 to 8 weeks.[39] Generally, more acute cases are treated more aggressively, receiving several sessions per week. Treatment of chronic cases is typically performed weekly for 3 to 4 sessions usually followed by tapering of frequency to once monthly or on an as-needed basis.[40] A recent meta-analysis of 23 human acupuncture studies (3461 patients) showed that short duration

($\leq$30 minutes), less frequent (twice weekly or less) acupuncture sessions yield long-lasting effects.[41]

Clinical Application of Acupuncture in Equine Practice

When applying a TCVM approach in the treatment of equine clinical conditions, a pattern diagnosis is paramount for most effective treatment.[42] However, there are many commonly used local and distal acupoints, as well as acupoints with special indications, that may be beneficial and can be used independent of pattern diagnosis.[29] Therapeutic acupuncture points for common clinical conditions in horses are discussed below.

Cervical stiffness

Cervical stiffness is a common complaint among equine athletes that negatively affects performance.[43,44] Normal head and neck movement is important for the equine gait and balance. Abnormal movement of the neck results in a variety of presenting signs including resistance to turning, forelimb lameness, poor performance, and abnormal gait.[43] Depending on the underlying cause of cervical stiffness, neurologic abnormalities such as weakness and proprioceptive ataxia may manifest and pain is commonly present.[43] Acupuncture treatment has been shown to improve cervical stiffness and decrease pain in horses, and improve neurologic signs by at least one clinical grade in dogs.[43] Additionally, acupuncture is safe and inexpensive for use as a first-line singular therapy or in combination with conventional therapeutics.[6,43] On the acupuncture point scan, horses with cervical stiffness typically show the most sensitivity around affected cervical articular processes and surrounding musculature in the author's(EM) experience. Horses with severe pain or stiffness in the poll region may not allow scanning of the region. This behavior must be differentiated from head-shyness or ear-shyness unrelated to cervical pain.

Therapeutic acupuncture points for cervical stiffness.

- Top 10 points:
  - *Jing-jia-ji* (Dorsal and ventral paravertebral acupoints)
  - *Jiu-wei* (Cervical 9 acupoints)
  - SI-3, SI-4, LU-7, BL-10, GB-20, GB-21, LI-15, TH-3
- Other points:
  - LI-4, LI-16, LI-18
  - ST-9, ST-10
  - GB-44
  - BL-11, BL-60, BL-62, BL-67
  - TH-1, TH-5, TH-15, TH-16
  - SI-1, SI-3, SI-16
  - GV-16 (**Fig. 1**)

Back pain

Back pain is another common cause of decreased performance in equine athletes and encompasses a variety of pathologic conditions affecting the thoracolumbar, lumbosacral, and sacroiliac regions.[43] Proper use of the back is vital for power and maintenance of balance and gait, and back pain frequently presents with general pack of performance, undesirable behavior under saddle, and muscle atrophy of the topline. Independent of the underlying cause, acupuncture may provide pain relief and alleviate muscle spasms, allowing the horse to properly engage the back during exercise to strengthen muscles of spinal stabilization.[40,43] Multiple studies have found acupuncture effective for the treatment of chronic thoracolumbar pain.[7,8] Horses

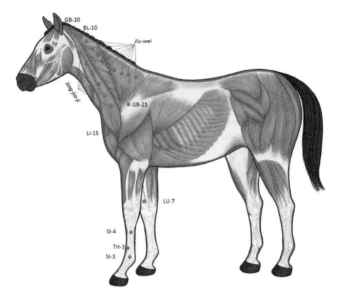

Fig. 1. Top acupoints for the treatment of cervical stiffness. (*From* H. Xie, Equine Acupuncture Chart, Chi University, Reddick, Florida, 2022.)

with back pain commonly show local sensitivity on acupuncture point scan of the Bladder and Governing Vessel meridians. Use of the horse, saddle fit, and rider ability can all impact comfort of the horse's back. Epaxial muscle soreness typically resolves with 1 to 3 acupuncture treatments. If minimal improvement is seen after 3 treatments, further diagnostics and conventional therapy may be required to diagnose a more significant underlying cause.

Therapeutic acupuncture points for thoracolumbar pain.

- Top 10 points:
  - BL-10, BL-11, BL-40, BL-65, BL-67
  - Two *Hua-tuo-jia-ji* (paravertebral) acupoints cranial and caudal to site of interest, or directly within locus of pain if horse is tolerant of needle placement
  - *Shen-shu, Shen-peng, Shen-jiao*
- Other points:
  - Bai-hui, GV-5, GV-6, GV-7
  - BL-23, BL-57, BL-60, and any BL points cranial and caudal to the locus of pain
  - LIV-3, LIV-13
  - GB-27, GB-34, GB-41, GB-44
  - KID-1
  - Yan-chi

Therapeutic acupuncture points for lumbosacral regional pain.

- Top 10 points:
  - Bai-hui
  - BL-23, and 2 BL acupoints cranial and caudal to the locus of pain
  - Shen-shu, Shen-peng, Yao-qian, Yao-zong, Yao-huo, Yan-chi
- Other points:
  - BL-27, BL-40, BL-51, BL-52, BL-54, BL-67

- ○ LIV-3, LIV-13
- ○ GB-34, GB-44

Therapeutic acupuncture acupoints for sacroiliac regional pain.

- • Top 10 points:
  - ○ Bai-hui, Shen-shu, Shen-peng, Shen-jiao, Wei-jian, Yan-chi
  - ○ Eight sacral acupoints (Ba-jiao)
  - ○ BL-53, BL-54, GB-27
- • Other points:
  - ○ BL-10, BL-11, BL-23, BL-27, BL-40, BL-51, BL-52, BL-67
  - ○ LIV-3, LIV-13
  - ○ GB-27, GB-34, GB-44
  - ○ GV-1, GV-2
  - ○ Yao-qian, Yao-zong, Yao-huo, Wei-gen (**Fig. 2**)

Colic

In the United States, colic remains the leading cause of death in horses from 1 to 20 years of age.[45] In TCVM, many types of colic are identified, including food stagnation, *Qi* stagnation, cold colic, and damp heat colic. Acupuncture may be used in medically or surgically managed colic cases to relieve pain, decrease spasms within the gastrointestinal tract, and improve gastrointestinal homeostasis.[46] Acupuncture may also decrease reflux volumes and improve appetite in the anorexic animal. Although more robust clinical trials are needed to evaluate the effects of acupuncture on gastrointestinal motility in equids, studies performed in other species have identified motility-normalizing effects.[47,48] In most cases, the underlying cause of colic must be addressed with conventional means. However, acupuncture may serve as a useful component of multimodal pain management and gastrointestinal prokinetic. The use of acupuncture for pain management is especially useful in horses where

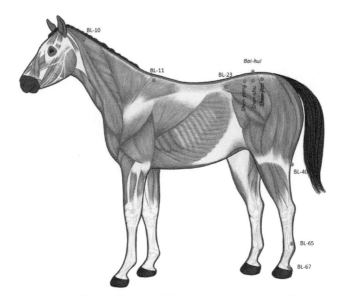

Fig. 2. Top acupoints for the treatment of back pain in the horse. (*From* H. Xie, Equine Acupuncture Chart, Chi University, Reddick, Florida, 2022.)

pharmaceutical options may be limited due to reduced renal or hepatic function and recent inconsistent opioid availability.

Therapeutic acupuncture points for colic.

- Top 10 points:
  - LI-11
  - BL-20, BL-21, BL-25
  - ST-2, ST-36, ST-37
  - *Jiang-ya, Bai-hui, Er-ding*
- Other points:
  - LI-4
  - LIV-3
  - ST-25, ST-40
  - SP-6, SP-9
  - GV-1, GV-4, GV-14, GV-26
  - CV-12 (**Fig. 3**)

Laminitis

Laminitis is a common complaint in all types of horses. In TCVM, laminitis is defined as *Qi* and/or blood stagnation at the feet and can be caused by excessive concussion to the feet, or internal injury, such as endotoxemia. The use of acupuncture to relieve pain is well-documented and spares the renal and hepatobiliary systems from the effects of chronic nonsteroidal anti-inflammatory drug administration.[11,12] Several studies have demonstrated the efficacy of acupuncture for the treatment of laminitis in horses and ponies.[49,50] In addition to pain management, acupuncture also functions to normalize perfusion and reduce formation of scar tissue, which may be beneficial in the laminitic horse.[40]

The distribution of sensitive acupoints in laminitis cases will be similar to horses with navicular syndrome or other foot-associated lameness but with greater severity.[6]

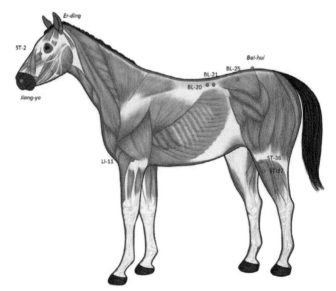

Fig. 3. Top acupoints for the treatment of colic in horses. (*From* H. Xie, Equine Acupuncture Chart, Chi University, Reddick, Florida, 2022.)

Sensitive acupoints include LI-18 and PC-1, with additional information provided by sensitivity at BL-13, BL-14, and BL-15, correlated to medial hoof, heel, and lateral hoof, respectively.

Therapeutic acupuncture points for forelimb laminitis.

- Top 10 points:
  - *Jing-well* points (TH-1, PC-9)
  - LI-3, LI-15
  - SI-3, SI-9
  - *Qian-ti-men*
  - LIV-3
  - BL-11, BL-18
- Other points:
  - *Jing-well* points (LU-11, LI-1, SI-1, HT-9)
  - BL-19
  - Bai-hui

Therapeutic acupuncture points for hind limb laminitis.

- Top 10 points:
  - *Jing-well* points (KID-1, ST-45)
  - GB-41, SP-3
  - BL-11, BL-18, BL-54, BL-65
  - *Hou-ti-men*
  - LIV-3
- Other points:
  - *Jing-well* points (SP-1, LIV-1, GB-44, BL-67)
  - BL-19
  - *Bai-hui, Shen-shu*

Therapeutic acupuncture points for acute laminitis.

- Use the described fore or hind limb laminitis points, with the addition of:
  - GV-14
  - *Qian-chan-wan, Xiong-tang, Hou-chan-wan, Qu-chi* (**Fig. 4**)

Laryngeal hemiplegia

Laryngeal hemiplegia, also known as recurrent laryngeal neuropathy (RLN), is a degenerative condition of the recurrent laryngeal nerve of horses that results in various degrees of laryngeal paralysis.[51] The inability to fully retract the arytenoid cartilage and vocal fold during inspiration creates the characteristic "roaring" noise heard during exercise.[51] In TCVM, RLN is characterized as deficiency of *Qi* and *Jing*.[16] The neuromodulatory effects of acupuncture, especially electroacupuncture, are useful in the restoration of laryngeal function in horses suffering from RLN.[16] Acupuncture is effective for restoration of function, with low-grade RLN (up to grade III) showing the highest success rates.[6,16] Positive response to acupuncture therapy is correlated with instituting acupuncture therapy quickly on identification of clinical signs in the acute phase of the condition.[16] Horses with RLN may not show sensitivity to acupuncture point scan.

Therapeutic acupuncture points for RLN.

- Top 10 points:
  - LU-7
  - LI-15, LI-17, LI-18

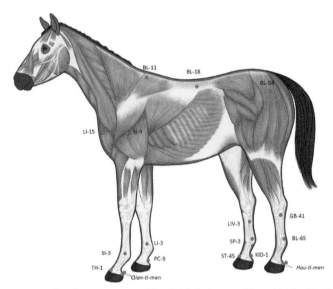

Fig. 4. Top acupoints for the treatment of laminitis in horses. (*From* H. Xie, Equine Acupuncture Chart, Chi University, Reddick, Florida, 2022.)

- o GB-21, CV-23, ST-9, SI-17
- o *Hou-bi, Hou-shu*
- Other points:
  - o LI-4, LI-10, LI-16
  - o ST-36
  - o SI-3
  - o KID-1, KID-3
  - o BL-20
  - o TH-17
  - o *Qi-hai-shu* (**Fig. 5**)

Suprascapular neuropathy (sweeney)

Suprascapular neuropathy is a traumatic injury, typically resulting from high-velocity collision with other horses or solid objects.[51] The resulting suprascapular neurologic dysfunction causes the affected limb to rotate at the shoulder during weight-bearing due to paresis of the supraspinatus and infraspinatus muscles, which normally stabilize the shoulder.[52] The suprascapular nerve may regenerate and horses can regain the use of the limb without therapy; however, the neurogenic muscle atrophy is typically permanent.

Therapeutic acupuncture points for suprascapular neuropathy.

- Top 10 points:
  - o *Gong-zi, Zhou-shu, Fei-men*
  - o LI-10, LI-15, LI-16
  - o HT-3
  - o SI-9
  - o KID-27
  - o TH-14
- Other points:

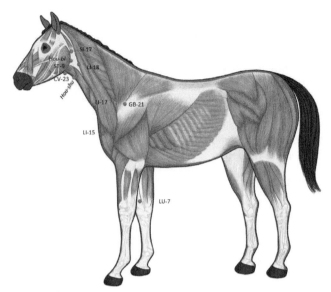

Fig. 5. Top acupoints for the treatment of laryngeal hemiplegia in horses. (*From* H. Xie, Equine Acupuncture Chart, Chi University, Reddick, Florida, 2022.)

- LI-1, LI-3, LI-4, LI-11
- SI-1, SI-3
- KID-24
- TH-1, TH-5, TH-9
- *Chong-tian*, *Fei-pan* (**Fig. 6**)

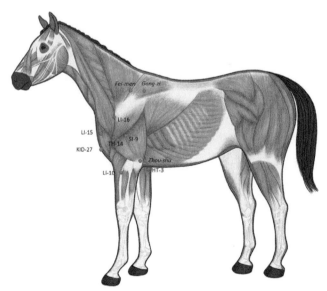

Fig. 6. Top acupoints for the treatment of suprascapular neuropathy in horses. (*From* H. Xie, Equine Acupuncture Chart, Chi University, Reddick, Florida, 2022.)

SUMMARY

Acupuncture has analgesic, neuromodulatory, and neuroregenerative effects, is inexpensive to provide, and does not rely on pharmaceutical administration. Acupuncture may aid the equine practitioner in the treatment of variety of musculoskeletal and internal medicine conditions including neck and back pain, colic, laminitis, laryngeal hemiplegia, suprascapular neuropathy, and nondiagnostic lameness, among many others. Although the evidence supporting the use of acupuncture for the treatment of various conditions is increasing, more double-blinded, placebo-controlled studies are required to strengthen the recommendation of acupuncture for the treatment of clinical conditions in the horse.

CLINICS CARE POINTS

- Acupuncture offers a non-invasive treatment for multiple conditions including spinal pain, laminitis, infertility, gastrointestinal disease, and laryngeal hemiplegia.
- Acupuncture has both local soft tissue and systemic effects on the body that contribute to its ability to provide pain relief, neurological recovery, and regulation of homeostasis.
- The most common forms of acupuncture include dry needle therapy, aquapunction (injection of pharmaceuticals), electroacupuncture, hemoacupuncture and moxibustion.
- Acupoints may be selected based upon a patient's TCVM pattern diagnosis, Western medical diagnosis, or a combination of both.

DISCLOSURE

The authors have no conflicts of interest to disclose.

REFERENCES

1. Yu C. Traditional Chinese veterinary acupuncture and Moxibustion. Beijing, China: China Agricultural Press; 1995.
2. Xie H, Chrisman C, Xie H, et al. Equine Acupuncture: From Ancient Art to Modern Validation. Am J Traditional Chin Vet Med 2009;4(2):1–4.
3. Shmalberg J, Memon MA. A Retrospective Analysis of 5,195 Patient Treatment Sessions in an Integrative Veterinary Medicine Service: Patient Characteristics, Presenting Complaints, and Therapeutic Interventions. Vet Med Int 2015;2015: 983621.
4. Memon MA, Sprunger LK. Survey of colleges and schools of veterinary medicine regarding education in complementary and alternative veterinary medicine. J Am Vet Med Assoc 2011;239(5):619–23.
5. Hunley S, Xie H. Veterinary Acupuncture: Current Use, Trends and Opinions - American Journal of Traditional Chinese Veterinary Medicine. Am J Traditional Vet Acupuncture 2011;6(2):55–62.
6. Xie H, Holyoak GR. Evidence-based Application of Acupuncture in Equine Practice. Am J Traditional Chin Vet Med 2021;16(2):41–52.
7. Xie H, Colahan P, Ott EA. Evaluation of electroacupuncture treatment of horses with signs of chronic thoracolumbar pain. J Am Vet Med Assoc 2005;227(2): 281–6.

8. Rungsri P, Trinarong C, Rojanasthien S. The effectiveness of electro-acupuncture on pain threshold in sport horses with back pain. Am J Traditional Chin Med 2009; 4(1):22–6.

9. Bello CA, Vianna AR, Nogueira K, et al. Acupuncture in the restoration of vaso-motor tonus of equine athletes with back pain. J Dairy Vet Anim Res 2018;7: 140–4.

10. Ying DW. Effect of Laser Acupuncture on Mitigating Anxiety in Acute Stressed Horses: A Randomized, Controlled Study. Am J Traditional Chin Med 2019; 14(1):33–40.

11. Faramarzi B, Lee D, May K, et al. Response to acupuncture treatment in horses with chronic laminitis. Can Vet J 2017;58(8):823.

12. Lee D, May, Faramarzi B. Comparison of First and Second Acupuncture Treat-ments in Horses with Chronic Laminitis. Iran J Vet Res 2019;20:9–12.

13. Aljobory AI, Jaafar S, Ahmed AS. Using acupuncture and electroacupuncture in the treatment of laminitis in racing horses: a comparative study. Coll Vet Med/Univ Mosul 2021;35(1):15–21.

14. Dunkel B, Pfau T, Fiske-Jackson A, et al. A pilot study of the effects of acupunc-ture treatment on objective and subjective gait parameters in horses. Vet Anaesth Analgesia 2017;44(1):154–62.

15. Thoresen S. Equine Sarcoid treated by acupuncture: eighteen cases. J Am Holist Vet Med Assoc 2018;50:75–80.

16. Kim M, Xie H. Use of electroacupuncture to treat laryngeal hemiplegia in horses. Vet Rec 2009;165(20):602.

17. Angeli AL, Luna SPL. Aquapuncture Improves Metabolic Capacity in Thorough-bred Horses. J Equine Vet Sci 2008;28(9):525–31.

18. Dewey CW, Xie H. The scientific basis of acupuncture for veterinary pain man-agement: A review based on relevant literature from the last two decades. Open Vet J 2021;11(2):203–9.

19. Alvarez L. Acupuncture. In: Gaynor J, Muir W, editors. Veterinary pain manage-ment. 3rd edition. St. Louis, MO: Elsevier; 2015. p. 365–79.

20. Pellegrini DZ, Müller TR, Fonteque JH, et al. Equine acupuncture methods and applications: A review. Equine Vet Educ 2020;32(5):268–77.

21. Yuan L, Mingxiao Y, Fan W, et al. Mechanism of electroacupuncture on inflamma-tory pain: neural-immune-endocrine interactions. JTCM 2019;39(50):740–9.

22. Lim HD, Kim KJ, Jo BG, et al. Acupuncture stimulation attenuates TNF-α produc-tion via vagal modulation in the concanavalin A model of hepatitis. Acupuncture Med 2020;38(6):417–25.

23. He JR, Yu SG, Tang Y, et al. Purinergic signaling as a basis of acupuncture-induced analgesia. Purinergic Signal 2020;16(3):297–304.

24. Ma SX. Nitric Oxide Signaling Molecules in Acupoints: Toward Mechanisms of Acupuncture. Chin J Integr Med 2017;23:812–5.

25. Melzack R, Stillwell DM, Fox EJ. Trigger points and acupuncture points for pain: Correlations and implications. Pain 1977;3(1):3–23.

26. Xie H, Wedemeyer L. The Validity of Acupuncture in Veterinary Medicine. Am J Traditional Chin Vet Med 2012;7(1):35–43.

27. Xie H, Sivula N. Review of Veterinary Acupuncture Clinical Trials. Am J Traditional Chin Vet Med 2017;11(1):35–46.

28. Roynard P, Frank L, Xie H, et al. Acupuncture for Small Animal Neurologic Disor-ders. Vet Clin North Am Small Anim Pract 2018;48(1):201–19.

29. Xie H, Preast V. Xie's veterinary acupuncture. Ames, IA: Blackwell Publishing; 2006.

30. Zhang GF, Huang Y, Tang CZ, et al. Characteristics of PET cerebral functional imaging during' Deqi' of acupuncture in healthy volunteers. Acupuncture Res 2011; 36(1):46–51.

31. Zhou W, Benharash P. Effects and Mechanisms of Acupuncture Based on the Principle of Meridians. J Acupuncture Meridian Stud 2014;7(4):190–3.

32. Maurer N, Nissel H, Egerbacher M, et al. Anatomical Evidence of Acupuncture Meridians in the Human Extracellular Matrix: Results from a Macroscopic and Microscopic Interdisciplinary Multicentre Study on Human Corpses. Evid Based Complement Altern Med 2019;2019:6976892.

33. Cheng KJ. Neuroanatomical Characteristics of Acupuncture Points: Relationship between Their Anatomical Locations and Traditional Clinical Indications. Acupuncture Med 2018;29(4):289–94.

34. Xie H, Wedemeyer L. Practical Guide to Traditional Chinese veterinary medicine: equine practice. Reddick, FL: Chi Institute Press; 2015.

35. Goe A, Shmalberg J, Gatson B, et al. Epinephrine or Gv-26 electrical stimulation reduces inhalant anesthestic recovery time in common snapping turtles (Chelydra Serpentina). J Zoo Wildl Med 2016;47(2):501–7.

36. Santos Godoi TLO, Villas-Boas JD, Almeida NA dos S, et al. Pharmacopuncture Versus Acepromazine in Stress Responses of Horses During Road Transport. J Equine Vet Sci 2014;34(2):294–301.

37. Pons A, Canfrán S, Benito J, et al. Effects of dexmedetomidine administered at acupuncture point GV20 compared to intramuscular route in dogs. J Small Anim Pract 2017;58(1):23–8.

38. le Jeune S. Prospective Study on the Correlation of Positive Acupuncture Scan and Lameness in 102 Performance Horses. Am J Traditional Chin Vet Med 2014;9(2):33–41.

39. Xie H, Holyoak GR. Tips to Improve Acupuncture Results for Lameness in Horses. In: American Association of Equine Practitioners Conference Proceedings. December 1-5 2018; San Francisico, CA.

40. le Jeune S, Henneman K, May K. Acupuncture and Equine Rehabilitation. Vet Clin Equine Pract 2016;32(1):73–85.

41. Chen YJ, Chen CT, Liu JY, et al. What Is the Appropriate Acupuncture Treatment Schedule for Chronic Pain? Review and Analysis of Randomized Controlled Trials. Evid Based Complement Altern Med 2019;2019:5281039.

42. Xie H. Black Box Theory and Diagnostic System of Traditional Chinese Veterinary Medicine. Am J Traditional Chin Vet Med 2017;12(1):1–5.

43. Pasteur CW. A Randomized, Controlled, Blinded Study of the Effectiveness of Acupuncture for Treatment of Cervical Stiffness in Horses. Am J Traditional Chin Vet Med 2021;16(1):1–10.

44. Pasteur CW. Review of Equine Cervical Pain. Am J Traditional Chin Vet Med 2016; 11(2):63–8.

45. *Equine Mortality in the United States*. USDA–APHIS–VS–CEAH–NAHMS. Available at: https://www.aphis.usda.gov. *Accessed* March 23, 2022.

46. Merritt AM, Xie H, Lester GD, et al. Evaluation of a method to experimentally induce colic in horses and the effects of acupuncture applied at the Guan-yuan-shu (similar to BL-21) acupoint. Am J Vet Res 2002;63(7):1006–11.

47. Wang JJ, Liu XD, Qin M, et al. Electro-acupuncture of Tsusanli and Shangchuhsu regulates gastric activity possibly through mediation of the vagus-solotary complex. Hepatogastroenterology 2007;54(78):1862–7.

48. Chen J, Song GQ, Yin J, et al. Electroacupuncture improves impaired gastric motility and slow waves induced by rectal distension in dogs. Am J Physiol Gastrointest Liver Physiol 2008;295(3):614–20.
49. Waguespack RW, Hanson DRR. Treating Navicular Syndrome in Equine Patients. Compend Contin Educ Vet 2011;33(1):2.
50. Lancaster LS, Bowker RM. Acupuncture Points of the Horse's Distal Thoracic Limb: A Neuroanatomic Approach to the Transposition of Traditional Points. Animals 2012;2:455–71.
51. Draper AC, Piercy RJ. Pathological classification of equine recurrent laryngeal neuropathy. J Vet Intern Med 2018;32(4):1397–409.
52. Emond AL, Bertoni L, Seignour M, et al. Peripheral neuropathy of a forelimb in horses: 27 cases (2000–2013). J Am Vet Med Assoc 2016;249(10):1187–95.

Clinical Application of Chinese Herbal Medicine in Equine Practice

Emily Mangan, DVM, CTCVMP, CCRV, CVMMP[a],*,
Huisheng Xie, DVM, MS, PhD[b]

KEYWORDS

• Equine • Integrative medicine • Herbal medicine • Chinese medicine • TCVM

KEY POINTS

• The use of Chinese herbal medicine in horses has been increasing during the last few decades in the United States and other countries.
• Evidence-based studies have demonstrated the efficacy of Chinese herbal medicine for the treatment of equine diseases, although further clinical research is necessary.
• Chinese Herbal medicine can be safely prescribed by educated equine practitioners and is well-tolerated in most horses.

INTRODUCTION

Traditional Chinese herbal medicine (CHM) is one of the oldest surviving ethnopharmacological systems in the world, with records documenting the use of CHM for the treatment of equine disease dating back at least 4000 years.[1] Although CHM, along with the other common traditional Chinese veterinary medicine (TCVM) modalities such as acupuncture, have been used for the treatment of injury and disease for millennia, the introduction to the Western world and application of the scientific process has been relatively recent within the last few decades.[1–4]

According to the World Health Organization (WHO), about 80% of the human global population currently relies on botanical medicine.[5] Within developed counties, about 50% of new pharmaceuticals are being developed from plant or fungal origins, including compounds for use in oncology, cardiology, internal medicine, anesthesia, and analgesia.[6] Pharmacologically active phytochemicals identified in herbal medicines include alkaloids, terpenoids, glycosides, phenolic compounds, and fatty acids.[7]

[a] Wisewood Integrative Veterinary Medicine, LLC, PO Box 608, Pleasant Hill, OR 97455, USA;
[b] Chi University, 9650 West Highway 318, Reddick, FL 32686, USA
* Corresponding author.
E-mail address: emilymanganDVM@gmail.com

Vet Clin Equine 38 (2022) 541–555
https://doi.org/10.1016/j.cveq.2022.06.009
0749-0739/22/© 2022 Elsevier Inc. All rights reserved.

Studies in equids and other domestic species have shown herbal formulas to be efficacious for the treatment of musculoskeletal,[8] neurological,[9] cardiac,[10] pulmonary,[7] gastrointestinal,[11] urological,[12] reproductive,[13] endocrine,[14] dermatologic,[15] oncological,[16] and immunological diseases.[17] This botanical knowledge, although contained within an alternate paradigm of medical reasoning, may provide a wealth of knowledge on which to draw for the treatment of a variety of clinical conditions in the horse.

CHM has gained popularity as a primary and integrative treatment modality within the human and veterinary medical fields, with the increasing use in equids paralleling the use in human medicine.[3,18] This growing interest in traditional Chinese medical modalities has served as an impetus for Western medical practitioners to seek continuing education in TCVM as well as bolster a growing body of researchers and clinical scientists dedicated to elucidating TCVM mechanisms and the clinical use of CHM in horses.[3,19]

EASTERN AND WESTERN PERSPECTIVES ON HERBAL MEDICINE

Traditional Chinese medicine is a distinct, complex, and self-referential medical system that relies on a series of principles developed from a Taoist observation of the known world.[20] These principles include the theory of *Yin* and *Yang*, which can be considered as the balance between 2 opposing forces, and the Five Elements, which was borne of observation of natural cycle of the terrestrial world.[20–22] Each herb has specific properties and indications, and each herbal medicine formulation has been devised for a specific purpose, often using several herbs for a complete and balanced medicine.[1,23] These formulations are called patent formulations, which are made from ancient recipes that specify the amount and type of each herb to be included, and may contain up to 20 herbs.[24] An example of herbal formulation is available is **Fig. 1**. Patent formulas are frequently sold by modern herbal manufacturers, although manufacturers may make substitutions to the original formulas. Patent formulas that have been altered will typically refer to the "classical antecedent," indicating which patent formula served as the basis for the modified formulation.[25]

The main difference between the Eastern and Western cultural perspective on ethnopharmacology is that TCVM focuses on the identification of the herb itself as medicine versus the conventional approach of identification and isolation of specific active compounds responsible for the reported biologic effects.[24] Examples include aspirin from the bark of the willow tree. The original identified compound within willow bark is salicylic acid, and has been synthetized as acetylsalicylic acid, which is more potent.[26] The discovery that the multicomponent aspect of the willow bark is important for the full range of biochemical effects is a good example of synergism of active components, and an example of the importance of evaluating the effects the whole herb.[24,26]

HERBAL DOSAGE AND USAGE

The dosage of herbal medicines depends on the patient, the disease being treated, and the form of herbal medicine available.[23] The typical dose for the average sized horse is 15 to 30 grams of loose powder administered orally twice daily as a topdressing on feed or by an oral dosing syringe[23] (**Table 1**). Treatment duration depends on resolution of clinical signs. If improvement in clinical signs is seen within 2 weeks after initiating herbal administration, then the administration is continued for another 4 to 8 weeks.[23] If the clinical condition resolves within 4 weeks, then the dose is typically reduced by 50%, and continued for another 4 weeks.[23]

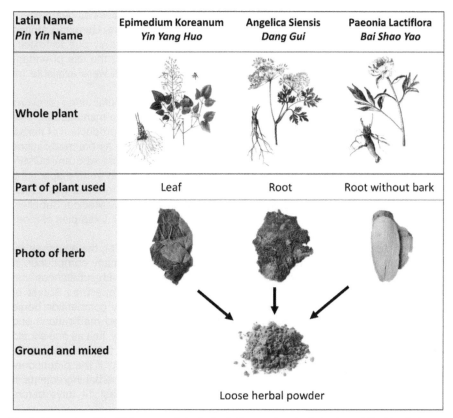

Latin Name *Pin Yin* Name	Epimedium Koreanum *Yin Yang Huo*	Angelica Siensis *Dang Gui*	Paeonia Lactiflora *Bai Shao Yao*
Whole plant			
Part of plant used	Leaf	Root	Root without bark
Photo of herb			
Ground and mixed		Loose herbal powder	

Fig. 1. Example of the Chinese medicinal plant, the used part of plant, and final herbal powder mixture of a formulation. These herbal ingredients are 3 of the 11 herbs in the patent formula *Zhuang Jin Jian Fang*.[23,25] Whole plant illustrations from Xie H, Preast V. *Xie's* Chinese Veterinary Herbology. Wiley-Blackwell 2010; with permission.

REGULATION AND LEGISLATION

Some of the most common controversies raised in the prescription or administration of herbal medicines are related to efficacy, safety, and quality control of the medications.[27] In the United States, many herbal medications fall under the jurisdiction of the Food and Drug Administration (FDA) and are considered dietary supplements, which

Table 1
Herbal medicine dosages for horses, ponies, and foals for raw powder and extract granules

Herbal Form	Species	Size	Dosage
Raw powder	Equine	Foal	Top dressing with food 3–8 g twice daily
		Pony	Top dressing with food 10–20 g, twice daily
		Horse	Top-dressing with food 15–30 g, twice daily
Extract granules (concentrated)	Equine	Foal	1–2 teaspoon, twice daily
		Pony	2–4 teaspoon, twice daily
		Horse	3–6 teaspoon, twice daily

Data from Ma A, ed. Clinical Manual of Chinese Veterinary Herbal Medicine. 5th ed. Ancient Art Press; 2020.

means that they do not undergo the same rigorous approval process as pharmaceuticals.[28,29] Several countries, including the United States, Canada, Germany, United Kingdom, and Israel have banned various herbal medicines, mainly due to toxicity (eg, herbs containing ephedrine, aristolochic acid, or aconite) or the use of endangered animal parts.[1,30] In countries where these banned herbs were available for use, they were not commonly prescribed.[1,30]

The FDA and the WHO provide references for current good manufacturing practices (cGMP), defined as a set of minimum requirements for facilities to manufacture, process, or a pack nutraceuticals or drugs, which are applied to the production of herbal medicines.[31-33] Current recommendations are to only purchase herbal medications from reputable sources who follow cGMP. Herbal manufacturers who are cGMP-compliant will typically advertise their status, and practitioners may verify inspections via the FDA database. Examples of herbal medicine manufacturers that this author uses include Dr Xie's Jing Tang Herbal, Inc,[34] Evergreen Herb & Medical Supplies, LLC,[35] Kan Herb Company,[36] and Mayway Corporation[37] (**Box 1**). Examples of modern herbal products can be seen in **Fig. 2**.

Although there may be a clinical benefit to the utilization of CHM, the equine practitioner must be aware when treating competition horses that many compounds in herbal formulas are either directly testable or may cross-react with substances that are prohibited or banned by the International Federation for Equestrian Sports or the United States Equestrian Federation.[38,39] When treating any competition horse with herbal medicine, the practitioner must be aware of banned medications and medication withdrawal times set by the respective governing body, just as one should be aware when prescribing pharmaceuticals. Proprietary herbal formulas, where ingredients are not readily available, should be avoided. Similarly, if the practitioner cannot verify what metabolites are generated from the various herbal ingredients in a formula, the herbal medicines should be discontinued at least 14 days before competition.

SAFETY AND ADVERSITY

When prescribed appropriately, most readily available CHMs manufactured by reputable sources are safe for use in horses.[1,23] The most commonly observed adverse effect is self-limiting soft manure, which resolves within 1 to 3 days of discontinuation of the herbal medicine administration.[1] However, even though CHMs are not currently regulated as drugs in the United States, they should be treated with the same respect

---

Box 1
Selected list of reputable herbal manufacturers

Dr Xie's Jing Tang Herbal, Inc
  Website: www.tcvmherbal.com Phone: (800) 891-1986 Location: Ocala, FL

Evergreen Herbs & Medical Supplies, LLC
  Website: www.evherbs.com Phone: (866) 473-3697 Location: City of Industry, CA

Kan Herb Company
  Website: www.kanherb.com Phone: (831) 438-9450 Location: Santa Cruz, CA

Mayway Corporation
  Website: www.mayway.com Phone: (800) 262-9929 Location: Oakland, CA

Data from Refs.[34-37]

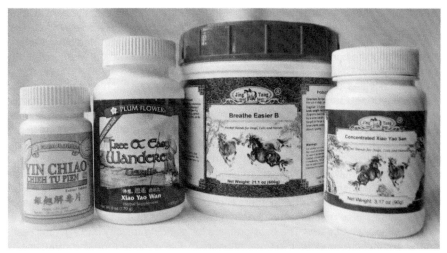

Fig. 2. Common formulations of herbal medicine, including *Yin Chiao Chieh Tu Pien* in the form of a compressed tablet, *Xiao Yao Wan* in the form of a tea pill, Breath Easier B (classical antecedent *Ge Jie San*) in the form of loose herbal powder, and concentrated *Xiao Yao San* in the form of concentrated granules. Photos of herbal products from Mayway Corporation and Dr Xie's Jing Tang Herbal, Inc used with permission.

as pharmaceuticals by equine practitioners.[1] As herbal formulas become more readily available, reports of adverse reactions have also increased, highlighting the importance of education and proper prescription of these medicines to reduce the incidence of toxicity and adverse reactions.[1,3] The most common causes of Chinese herbal toxicity include toxic properties of individual herbs, improper substitution of herbs in formulas, improper combination of herbs in formulas, improper herb extraction and processing techniques, overdosing, inappropriate long-term use, interactions with conventional pharmaceuticals, individual sensitivity to medications, and incorrect TCVM pattern diagnosis.[1]

For example, any herb containing aconitine (such as Aconite *Fu Zi*) can be neurotoxic.[1] The herb Akebia *Mu Tong* is safe but may be wrongly substituted with Aristolochia *Guan Mu Tong*, which contains aristolochic acid and can cause life-threatening nephrotoxicity.[1] Armeniaca *Ku Xing Ren* and Persica *Tao Ren* both contain amygdalin and when combined in a single formula, the amount of amygdalin and hydrocyanic acid effectively doubles as shown with quantization toxicology, which makes an herbal formula containing these 2 herbs toxic.[1] Raw (unprocessed) Aconite root *Fu Zi* contains high concentrations of aconitine but the aconitine is easily hydrolyzed to a mildly toxic alkaline when prepared with the traditional decoction process of boiling and heating.[1]

These forms of toxicity occur at the manufacturer level and can be avoided by obtaining herbal medicines from reputable manufacturers that publish their ingredients and ingredient sources.[1] Similarly, toxicity at the practitioner level, including adverse events related to overdosing, inappropriate length of administration, or incorrect TCVM pattern diagnosis, can be avoided with practitioner education on the appropriate use of herbal medicines.[1]

In contrast to the common misconception that there is little available literature on the safety of CHM, more than 12,800 herbs have been studied, and information regarding toxicities, cautions and precautions, contraindications, and incompatibilities are well-documented.[40] Reputable literature for practitioners looking to prescribe herbal medicines include Xie's Chinese Veterinary Herbology,[23] Clinical Manual of Chinese Veterinary Herbal Medicine,[25] Chinese Herbal Medicine: Materia Medica,[41] and the herbal database "About Herbs" available from the Memorial Sloan Kettering Cancer Center.[42]

Known toxicities of CHM include cardiovascular toxicity, such as ephedrine and pseudoephedrine found in Ephedra *Ma Huang*, nephrotoxicity due to aristolochic acid found in Aristolochia *Guan Ma Tong*, neurotoxicity due to aconite found in Aconite *Chuan Wu*, and hepatotoxicity from several herbs, including Melia *Chuan Lian Zi*.[1,30] Some of these herbs (such as Ephedra) are banned and are not used in herbal formulas in the West,[30] and other herbs that may have hepatotoxic properties may be used in small quantities with the recommendation of monitoring of liver function tests on serum biochemistry profiles.[1]

As the use of CHM is increasing, there is great need for the continuation of research into herbal medicine mechanisms of action and scientific characterization of their reported therapeutic effects.[1] The best practice for avoiding toxicity and adverse reactions is continuing education for practitioners in CHM, careful dosing, and use of products produced from cGMP facilities.[1]

CLINICAL APPLICATIONS

For best outcome in the clinical patient, correct TCVM pattern diagnosis is paramount for appropriate herbal medicine selection.[1] However, herbal medicine may still be effective when prescribed based on Western clinical signs and offers the equine practitioner an additional modality as primary treatment of mild disease or financially constrained cases, or as a complementary therapy for refractory or severe injury or disease. A summary of clinical conditions and herbal medicines is available in **Table 2**.

Tendon and Ligament Injuries

Tendon and ligament injuries are common in equine athletes and may result in long layups or loss of use of the animal for the intended discipline.[43] CHM may be used as a primary treatment of mild tendon or ligament injuries or empirical treatment of suspected injuries in cases where definitive diagnosis is cost-prohibitive or otherwise restricted, as well as a complementary therapy for horses undergoing other therapies. Although some injuries are easily accessible for diagnostic imaging and treatment with platelet rich plasma, stem cells, extracorporeal shockwave, low-level laser, or acupuncture, other tendinous or ligamentous structures of the spine, pelvis, or within the hoof capsule are more difficult to image or provide direct medical intervention.

In TCVM, tendon and ligaments are governed by the Wood element and are typically seen in horses with Wood personalities (eg, hard worker, aggressive, wants to lead), which describe the majority of racing thoroughbreds and warmbloods.[22,43] The Wood element is most affected in the spring and is dominant in young animals.[22] The chosen herbal formula should nourish the tendons and ligaments and clear inflammation and pain. CHM recommendations for tendon and ligament injures include the following:

- Angelica *Dang Gui* or *Zhuang Jin Jian Fang* at 15 grams by mouth twice daily until healed.
- Topical application of *Zhi Tong Gao* to the affected structure once daily.[25]

Navicular Syndrome

Navicular syndrome is characterized by chronic, progressive forelimb lameness due to caudal heel pain and associated degeneration of the navicular bone and

Table 2
Herbal medicines listed by clinical conditions in equids

Clinical Condition	Chinese Herbal Medicine
Tendon or ligament injury	• Angelica *Dang Gui* or *Zhuang Jin Jian Fang* at 15 g by mouth twice daily until healed • Topical application of *Zhi Tong Gao* to the affected structure once daily[25]
Navicular syndrome	• Oral *Sang Zhi San* at the standard dose of 15 g by mouth twice daily • Topical *Si Sheng San*, applied to the caudal heel once daily for no more than 2 weeks[25]

Laminitis	• Acute laminitis[25]
	  ○ *Yin Chen San* at 15–30 g by mouth twice daily
	• Acute flare-up of chronic laminitis[25]
	  ○ *Hong Hua San* at 15 g by mouth twice daily until resolution
	• Chronic laminitis[25]
	  ○ Modified *Jin Gui Shen Qi* at 15 g by mouth twice daily

Chronic diarrhea	• Chronic diarrhea containing undigested feed[25]
	  ○ *Shen Ling Bai Zhu* at 15 g by mouth twice daily until resolution
	• Prolonged diarrhea in geriatric horses[25]
	  ○ *Si Shen Wan* at 15 g by mouth twice daily until resolution

Gastric ulceration	• Mild cases of gastric ulceration[25]
	  ○ *Wei Le San* at 15 g by mouth twice daily until resolution
	• Severe cases of gastric ulceration[25]
	  ○ *Yu Nu Jian* at 15 g by mouth twice daily until resolution

Equine asthma	• Seasonal acute equine asthma[25]
	  ○ Schisandra 5 at 15 g by mouth twice daily until resolution
	• Equine asthma with dry cough[25]
	  ○ *Bai He Gu Jin* at 15 g by mouth twice daily until resolution
	• Equine asthma with weak cough and generalized weakness[25]
	  ○ *Bu Fei San* at 15 g by mouth twice daily until resolution
	• Severe equine asthma with wheezing[25]
	  ○ *Hu Xi Chang* at 15 g by mouth twice daily until resolution

Exercise-induced pulmonary hemorrhage	• Single Immortal B at 30 g by mouth twice daily 3 days before racing and 3 days after racing[25] • If EIPH is refractory to Single Immortal B, use *Bao Fei San* at 30 g by mouth twice daily 3 days before racing and 3 days after racing[25] • If the EIPH is still refractory to *Bao Fei San*, then the dose of *Bao Fei San* may be increased to 60 g twice daily, for 3 days before racing and 3 days after[25] • *Yunnan Bai Yao* at 4 g by mouth every 12 hours starting 36 hours before the onset of strenuous exercise, for a total of 12 grams given over 3 administrations[25]
Anhidrosis	• New *Xiang Ru San* at 15 g by mouth twice daily until resolved[25]

surrounding soft tissue structures.[44] Although a variety of clinical management therapeutics exist, including corrective farriery, pharmaceuticals, or surgical interventions, most horses will eventually become refractory to therapy as the degeneration progresses.[44]

CHM has been shown to decrease inflammation[45] and relieve pain.[46] Although high-quality studies in naturally occurring equine navicular syndrome are needed, this author has found success in utilizing the anti-inflammatory properties of CHM to relieve pain and reduce the reliance on nonsteroidal anti-inflammatory drugs (NSAIDs). The recommended herbal formulas for navicular syndrome include the following:

- Oral *Sang Zhi San* at the standard dose of 15 grams by mouth twice daily.
- Topical *Si Sheng San*, applied to the caudal heel once daily for no more than 2 weeks.[25]

Laminitis

Equine laminitis is degeneration of the junction between the horny and sensitive lamina of the hoof, and is a common sequala of equine metabolic syndrome, pars pituitary intermedia dysfunction, and endotoxicity.[47–49] Laminitis results in a characteristic lameness and posture, and diagnosis is typically made by clinical signs and physical examination in conjunction with diagnostic imaging.[49,50]

For best practices, herbal medicine should be used in combination with dietary management, use of soft footing, ice boots, and corrective farriery, along with diagnosis and appropriate management of any underlying endocrinopathies.[49] As CHM possesses anti-inflammatory properties,[45] administration of CHM may decrease the reliance on NSAID administration, which may be important in horses with comorbidities, such as renal or hepatic insufficiency. TCVM identifies 3 pattern diagnoses that result in the Western diagnosis of laminitis.[23]

- Acute laminitis[25]
  - Pattern diagnosis: Hot hooves, acutely painful. Red tongue. Fast pulse.
  - Herbal formula: *Yin Chen San* at 15 grams by mouth twice daily. If severe (Obel grade 3 or 4), then 30 grams by mouth twice daily may be given for up to 14 days before reducing dose to standard 15 grams by mouth twice daily.
- Acute flare-up of chronic laminitis[25]
  - Pattern diagnosis: Chronic laminitis with acute flare. Red tongue. Fast pulse.
  - Herbal formula: *Hong Hua San* at 15 grams by mouth twice daily until resolution.
- Chronic laminitis[25]
  - Pattern diagnosis: Chronic laminitis associated with equine metabolic syndrome or Cushing disease. Pale tongue. Weak pulse.
  - Herbal formula: Modified *Jin Gui Shen Qi* at 15 grams by mouth twice daily as maintenance.

Chronic Diarrhea

Chronic diarrhea or colitis in adult horses is frequently due to intestinal dysbiosis.[51] Antibiotic therapy is often implicated, and the administration of additional antibiotics is typically ineffectual and may worsen diarrheal diseases due to further disruption of beneficial commensal bacteria.[51] Current recommended therapies are nonspecific and mainly consist of supportive care to limit dehydration, inflammation, endotoxemia, laminitis, and coagulopathy, as well as probiotics and prebiotics to reestablish the gastrointestinal microbiome.[51]

CHM has been shown to be effective at promoting villus growth of gastric enterocytes, regulating gastric pH, and enhancing intestinal reepithelialization in mice.[52] More equine-specific studies are needed but as the effect of CHM is often conserved between species, CHM may provide benefit in refractory cases of chronic diarrhea in horses.

- Chronic diarrhea containing undigested feed[25]
  - Pattern diagnosis: Chronic diarrhea containing undigested feed, anorexia, and weight loss. Exercise tolerance. Pale tongue. Weak and deep pulse.

- o Herbal formula: *Shen Ling Bai Zhu* at 15 grams by mouth twice daily until resolution.
- Prolonged diarrhea in geriatric horses[25]
  - o Pattern diagnosis: Chronic diarrhea, mostly seen at night or early in the morning, cold and painful in the back, and stiff and weak pelvic limbs. Pale tongue. Weak and deep pulse.
  - o Herbal formula: *Si Shen Wan* at 15 grams by mouth twice daily until resolution.

Gastric Ulceration

Equine squamous gastric disease and equine glandular gastric disease are both common clinical conditions affecting performance horses.[53] Diagnosis by gastroscopy is standard, and treatment typically consists of diet, management, and husbandry changes, along with proton pump inhibitors or H_2-receptor agonists.[54]

CHM has been found effective in rats to improve healing of gastric mucosal injury,[55] and antibacterial against *Helicobacter pylori*, which commonly affects humans.[56] In experimentally induced gastric ulceration in horses, no effect between control and CHM treatment groups were observed.[57] However, it is important to consider that TCVM functions to treat imbalances in the body, and that experimentally induced injury is a different pattern diagnosis than a naturally occurring disease. More high-quality equine clinical studies of CHM treatment of naturally occurring gastric ulceration are required for evidence-based recommendation of CHM for this disease. Currently, recommendations for herbal use can only be in conjunction with established conventional treatment protocols. In TCVM, gastric ulcers are due to Heat in the Stomach and herbal formulas used to clear Stomach Heat include the following:

- For mild cases of gastric ulceration[25]
  - o Herbal formula: *Wei Le San* at 15 grams by mouth twice daily until resolution.
- For severe cases of gastric ulceration[25]
  - o Herbal formula: *Yu Nu Jian* at 15 grams by mouth twice daily until resolution.

Equine Asthma

Equine asthma is an allergic respiratory disease of the horse characterized by bronchoconstriction and mucus production, with increased exhalatory respiratory effort and tachypnea.[7,58] Treatment typically consists of environmental management, corticosteroids, bronchodilators, and mucolytics.[58]

Extracts of CHM compounds have been found to decrease infiltration of eosinophils in human asthmatics, downregulate the production of inflammatory cytokines, and inhibit nitric oxide production, which may mitigate early inflammatory pathways.[7] TCVM identifies 4 pattern diagnoses, with an herbal recommendation for each:

- Seasonal acute equine asthma[25]
  - o Pattern diagnosis: Clinical signs worsen in the summer or warm seasons, possible hives. Tongue is red and dry. Pulse is strong and fast.
  - o Herbal formula: Schisandra 5 at 15 grams by mouth twice daily until resolution.
- Equine asthma with dry cough[25]
  - o Pattern diagnosis: Dry cough, dry hair coat. Tongue is red and dry. Pulse is rapid.
  - o Herbal formula: *Bai He Gu Jin* at 15 grams by mouth twice daily until resolution.
- Equine asthma with weak cough and generalized weakness[25]
  - o Pattern diagnosis: Chronic disease, weak cough, fatigue. Tongue is pale and wet. Pulse is weak and deep.
  - o Herbal formula: *Bu Fei San* at 15 grams by mouth twice daily until resolution.

- Severe equine asthma with wheezing[25]
  - Pattern diagnosis: Chronic disease, hypertrophy of external abdominal obliques, wheezing, prolonged expiration. Tongue is pale with a thin coating. Pulse is weak and deep.
  - Herbal formula: *Hu Xi Chang* at 15 grams by mouth twice daily until resolution.

Exercise-Induced Pulmonary Hemorrhage

Exercise-induced pulmonary hemorrhage (EIPH) is bleeding that occurs in the lungs secondary to strenuous exercise and results in poor performance.[59] Only about 5% of horses with EIPH exhibit epistaxis, which is why diagnosis via endoscopic visualization or bronchoalveolar lavage is paramount for accurate diagnosis.[59] Furosemide is commonly prescribed preexercise to reduce the incidence of a severe hemorrhagic episode.[59]

In Chinese medicine, EIPH is due to Liver *Qi* Stagnation generating Heat, which is released through respiratory system as hemorrhage.[23] Three herbal formulas are indicated for EIPH: *Yunnan Bai Yao* (well-known for its hemostatic properties), Single Immortal B, and *Bao Fei San*.[23,25] *Yunnan Bai Yao* has been shown to decrease blood loss in elective ovariohysterectomies in dogs,[60] and Single Immortal B has been specifically formulated to clear heat and prevent bleeding.[25]

- Single Immortal B is the first line of CHM treatment, given 30 grams by mouth twice daily 3 days before racing and 3 days after racing.[25]
- If EIPH is refractory to Single Immortal B, then *Bao Fei San* may be used at the same dosing schedule of 30 grams by mouth twice daily 3 days before racing and 3 days after racing.[25]
- If the EIPH is still refractory to *Bao Fei San*, then the dose of *Bao Fei San* may be increased to 60 grams twice daily, for 3 days before racing and 3 days after.[25]
- *Yunnan Bai Yao* may be utilized for cases of EIPH that are continually refractory to Single Immortal B and *Bao Fei San* because some horses may still respond favorably to *Yunnan Bai Yao*. Administer 4 grams by mouth every 12 hours starting 36 hours before the onset of strenuous exercise, for a total of 12 grams given over 3 administrations.[25]

Anhidrosis

Anhidrosis is the inadequate production of sweat in response to elevated body temperature and affects approximately 2% to 6% of horses worldwide.[61,62] There is no clinically effective conventional treatment, although a wide variety of supplements exist on the market with limited and varying efficacy.[61–63] As such, alternative therapies, including acupuncture and herbal medicine, have become a mainstay of anhidrosis treatment modalities.[18,61,64,65]

The most common herbal medicine prescribed for anhidrosis is New *Xiang Ru San*, which is formulated to clear heat from the body.[23,25] The best time to initiate herbal medicine administration for the prevention of anhidrosis is in the springtime, before the true heat of summer. Treatment may be discontinued in the wintertime, once clinical signs have resolved. Practitioners should be aware that herbal medicine may mediate clinical signs but typically must be administered every summer as a management strategy. For the average size horse, the dose of New *Xiang Ru San* is as follows:

- New *Xiang Ru San* is administered at 15 grams by mouth twice daily until resolved.

SUMMARY

Traditional CHM has been practiced for around 4000 years and has been growing in popularity in North America and elsewhere for the last few decades. CHM exists within a complex, self-referential ethnobotanical system of TCVM, which may provide a wealth of knowledge for the equine practitioner and clinical researcher alike. The Chinese herbal medicine Materia Medica contains vast information about indications and contraindications of herbal medicines, elucidated by practitioners over thousands of years.[23,41] Although there is a growing body of evidence for the use of CHM, there is still a great need for high-quality, randomized, double-blinded placebo-controlled clinical studies in naturally occurring disease. Currently, herbal medicine is best indicated as an integrative or complementary modality, alongside conventional therapies for common equine diseases and injuries, although CHM may be safely used as a first-line of therapy in mild conditions, or as an additional modality for challenging, refractory cases.

CLINICS CARE POINTS

- Selection of Chinese herbal medicine is best made within the philosophical framework of Traditional Chinese veterinary medicine, although practitioners can successfully prescribe herbal medicine based on Western diagnoses.

- Herbal medicines are regulated as food supplements, not pharmaceuticals, and should only be purchased from reputable manufacturers in Food and Drug Administration-approved facilities that adhere to current good manufacturing practice guidelines.

- The most commonly observed adverse effect of Chinese herbal medicines is a loose manure. If this occurs, immediate discontinuation of the herbal medicine typically results in resolution of loose manure within 1 to 3 days.

- Some herbal medicines may contain or cross-react with testable prohibited or banned substances, so be mindful of prescription of herbal medicines in competition horses.

DISCLOSURE

Dr E. Mangan has no conflicts of interest to disclose while Dr H. Xie discloses that he is a co-owner of Dr Xie's Jing Tang Herbal, Inc.

REFERENCES

1. Xie H. Toxicity of Chinese veterinary herbal medicines. Am J Tradit Chin Vet Med 2011;6(2):10.
2. Xie H. Chinese veterinary herbal medicine: history, scientific validation and regulations. Am J Tradit Chin Vet Med 2012;7(1):5.
3. Schoen AM. Results of a survey on educational and research programs in complementary and alternative veterinary medicine at veterinary medical schools in the United States. J Am Vet Med Assoc 2000;216(4):502–9.
4. Marziani JA. Nontraditional therapies (traditional Chinese veterinary medicine and chiropractic) in exotic animals. Veterinary Clin North Am Exot Anim Pract 2018;21(2):511–28.
5. World Health Organization. WHO global report on traditional and complementary medicine 2019. World Health Organization; 2019. Available at: https://apps.who.int/iris/handle/10665/312342. Accessed March 23, 2022.

6. Newman DJ, Cragg GM. Natural products as sources of new drugs over the 30 years from 1981 to 2010. J Nat Prod 2012;75(3):311–35.
7. Tangjitjaroen W, Xie H, Colahan PT. The therapeutic actions of traditional Chinese herbal medicine used for the treatment of equine respiratory diseases. Am J Tradit Chin Vet Med 2009;4(1):7–21.
8. Arnold MD, Thornbrough LM. Treatment of musculoskeletal pain with traditional Chinese herbal medicine. Phys Med Rehabil Clin N Am 1999;10(3):663–71.
9. Cahyono T. Acupuncture for neurological disease unresponsive to western medications in 94 small animal cases. Am J Tradit Chin Vet Med 2015;10(2):19.
10. Zhao P, Su G, Xiao X, et al. Chinese medicinal herb Radix Astragali suppresses cardiac contractile dysfunction and inflammation in a rat model of autoimmune myocarditis. Toxicol Lett 2008;182(1):29–35.
11. Xie H, Liu H, Merritt AM, et al. Equine chronic diarrhea: traditional Chinese veterinary medicine review. J Equine Vet Sci 1997;17(12):667–74.
12. Raditic DM. Complementary and integrative therapies for lower urinary tract diseases. Vet Clin North Am Small Anim Pract 2015;45(4):857–78.
13. Huang X, Wang S, Wang L, et al. Administration of an herbal powder based on traditional Chinese veterinary medicine enhanced the fertility of Holstein dairy cows affected with retained placenta. Theriogenology 2018;121:67–71.
14. Wilcox DL, Liu H, Ma Y, et al. Comparison of the Chinese herbal formula Hai Zao Yu Hu Tang and methimazole for the treatment of feline hyperthyroidism. Am J Tradit Chin Vet Med 2009;4(1):27–38.
15. Gu SX, Zhang AL, Coyle ME, et al. Chinese herbal medicine for atopic eczema: an overview of clinical evidence. J Dermatolog Treat 2017;28(3):246–50.
16. Feng BB, Zhang JH, Xu XY, et al. Mechanisms of action of Chinese herbal medicines in the prevention and treatment of cancer. Am J Tradit Chin Vet Med 2010; 5(1):37–47.
17. Song D, Song J, Song X. Traditional Chinese veterinary medicine immunology and its application in the treatment of canine and feline diseases. Am J Tradit Chin Vet Med 2008;3(1):24–30.
18. Liu JJ, Memon MA, Ma A, et al. Prevalence, clinical features and Chinese herbal medicine prescription patterns of equine patients treated in a veterinary teaching hospital with traditional Chinese veterinary medicine: A retrospective study. Am J Tradit Chin Vet Med 2019;14(2):45–54.
19. Memon MA, Shmalberg J, Adair HS, et al. Integrative veterinary medical education and consensus guidelines for an integrative veterinary medicine curriculum within veterinary colleges. Open Vet J 2016;6(1):44–56.
20. Gu S, Pei J. Innovating Chinese herbal medicine: from traditional health practice to scientific drug discovery. Front Pharmacol 2017;8:381.
21. Xie H, Wedemeyer L, Chrisman CL, et al. Practical guide to traditional Chinese veterinary medicine: equine practice. Reddick, FL: Chi Institute Press; 2015.
22. Xie H. Xie's 2 W diagnostic system: using "where" and "what" in TCVM diagnostics. Am J Tradit Chin Vet Med 2016;11(1):16.
23. Xie H, Preast V. Xie's Chinese veterinary herbology. Ames, IA: Wiley-Blackwell; 2010.
24. Zhou X, Seto SW, Chang D, et al. Synergistic effects of Chinese herbal medicine: a comprehensive review of methodology and current research. Front Pharmacol 2016;7:1–16.
25. Ma A, editor. Clinical manual of Chinese veterinary herbal medicine. 5th edition. Gainesville, FL: Ancient Art Press; 2020.

26. Vlachojannis J, Magora F, Chrubasik S. Willow species and aspirin: different mechanism of actions. Phytother Res PTR 2011;25(7):1102–4.

27. Fan TP, Deal G, Koo HL, et al. Future development of global regulations of Chinese herbal products. J Ethnopharmacol 2012;140(3):568–86.

28. Suh Y. The regulation of Chinese medicine in the U.S. Longhua Chin Med 2020; 3(0):1–11.

29. Food and Drug Administration. Complementary and alternative medicine products and their regulation. 2020. Available at: https://www.fda.gov/regulatory-information/search-fda-guidance-documents/complementary-and-alternative-medicine-products-and-their-regulation-food-and-drug-administration. Accessed March 26, 2022.

30. Fleischer T, Su YC, Lin SJS. How do government regulations influence the ability to practice Chinese herbal medicine in Western countries. J Ethnopharmacol 2017;196:104–9.

31. WHO Expert Committee on Specifications for Pharmaceutical Preparations. Annex 2 Guidelines on Good Manufacturing Practices for the Manufacture of Herbal Medicines. 2018. Available at: https://www.who.int/traditional-complementary-integrative-medicine/publications/trs1010_annex2.pdf?ua=1. Accessed March 23, 2022.

32. U.S. Department of Health and Human Services, Food and Drug Administration. Silver Spring, MD: Botanical Drug Development Guidance for Industry; 2016. p. 34.

33. WHO Expert Committee on Specifications for Pharmaceutical Preparations. Annex 1 WHO Guidelines on Good Herbal Processing Practices for Herbal Medicines. 2018. Available at: https://www.who.int/traditional-complementary-integrative-medicine/publications/trs1010_annex1.pdf?ua=1. Accessed March 23, 2022.

34. Dr. Xie's Jing Tang Herbal, Inc. Available at: https://www.tcvmherbal.com/. Accessed June 15, 2022.

35. Evergreen Herbs & Medical Supplies, LLC. Available at: https://www.evherbs.com/. Accessed June 15, 2022.

36. Kan Herb Company. Available at: https://www.kanherb.com/. Accessed June 15, 2022.

37. Mayway Corporation. Available at: https://www.mayway.com/. Accessed June 15, 2022.

38. United States Equestrian Federation. 2022 USEF guidelines & rules for drugs and medications. 2022. Available at: https://www.usef.org/forms-pubs/2Zp2C_YKs4s/drugs-medications-guidelines. Accessed March 9, 2022.

39. Fédération Equestre Internationale (FEI). FEI warning regarding the administration of supplements to horses. 2021. Available at: https://inside.fei.org/system/files/FEI%20Warning%20re%20Supplement%20Use%20-%2019%20December%202015_0_0.pdf. Accessed March 9, 2022.

40. Leung AY. Traditional toxicity documentation of Chinese Materia Medica–an overview. Toxicol Pathol 2006;34(4):319–26.

41. Bensky D, Clavey S, Stöger E, et al. Chinese herbal medicine: meteria Medica. 3rd edition. Seattle, WA: Eastland Press; 2015.

42. Integrative Medicine: Search About Herbs | Memorial Sloan Kettering Cancer Center. Available at: https://www.mskcc.org/cancer-care/diagnosis-treatment/symptom-management/integrative-medicine/herbs/search. Accessed June 15, 2022.

43. Pasteur CW. Treatment of tendonitis in equines. Am J Tradit Chin Vet Med 2007; 2(1):4.

44. Osborn ML, Cornille JL, Blas-Machado U, et al. The equine navicular apparatus as a premier enthesis organ: functional implications. Vet Surg 2021;50(4):713–28.

45. Muluye RA, Bian Y, Alemu PN. Anti-inflammatory and antimicrobial effects of heat-clearing Chinese herbs: a current review. J Tradit Complement Med 2014; 4(2):93–8.

46. He DY, Dai SM. Anti-Inflammatory and Immunomodulatory Effects of Paeonia Lactiflora Pall., a Traditional Chinese Herbal Medicine. Front Pharmacol 2011;2. Available at: https://www.frontiersin.org/article/10.3389/fphar.2011.00010. Accessed March 26, 2022.

47. Lankenau CJ. Efficacy of Wu Mei Wan for treating equine metabolic syndrome related laminitis and uveitis poorly responsive to conventional medicine. Am J Tradit Chin Vet Med 2019;14(2):14.

48. de Laat MA, Sillence MN, Reiche DB. Phenotypic, hormonal, and clinical characteristics of equine endocrinopathic laminitis. J Vet Intern Med 2019;33(3): 1456–63.

49. Mitchell CF, Fugler LA, Eades SC. The management of equine acute laminitis. Vet Med Res Rep 2014;6:39–47.

50. Patterson-Kane JC, Karikoski NP, McGowan CM. Paradigm shifts in understanding equine laminitis. Vet J 2018;231:33–40.

51. McKinney CA, Oliveira BCM, Bedenice D, et al. The fecal microbiota of healthy donor horses and geriatric recipients undergoing fecal microbial transplantation for the treatment of diarrhea. PLoS One 2020;15(3):e0230148.

52. Zhang C, Ma A, Xie H. Review of clinical and experimental research from China on 8 Chinese herbal medicines for gastrointestinal disorders. Am J Tradit Chin Vet Med 2014;9:16.

53. Sykes BW, Bowen M, Habershon-Butcher JL, et al. Management factors and clinical implications of glandular and squamous gastric disease in horses. J Vet Intern Med 2019;33(1):233–40.

54. Sykes BW, Hewetson M, Hepburn RJ, et al. European college of equine internal medicine consensus statement—Equine Gastric Ulcer Syndrome in adult horses. J Vet Intern Med 2015;29(5):1288–99.

55. Yuan E, Liu L, Huang M, et al. Effects of complex extracts of traditional Chinese herbs on gastric mucosal injury in rats and potential underlying mechanism. Food Front 2021;2(3):305–15.

56. Li Y, Xu C, Zhang Q, et al. In vitro anti-Helicobacter pylori action of 30 Chinese herbal medicines used to treat ulcer diseases. J Ethnopharmacol 2005;98(3): 329–33.

57. Munsterman AS, Dias Moreira AS, Marqués FJ. Evaluation of a Chinese herbal supplement on equine squamous gastric disease and gastric fluid pH in mares. J Vet Intern Med 2019;33(5):2280–5.

58. Pirie RS. Recurrent airway obstruction: A review. Equine Vet J 2014;46(3):276–88.

59. Gold JR, Knowles DP, Coffey T, et al. Exercise-induced pulmonary hemorrhage in barrel racing horses in the Pacific Northwest region of the United States. J Vet Intern Med 2018;32(2):839–45.

60. Liu J, Ma A. A randomized, blinded, controlled study on the effects of preoperative oral administration of Yunnan Baiyao for the mitigation of blood loss in dogs undergoing elective spay/neuter surgeries. Am J Tradit Chin Vet Med 2020; 15(2):7–16.

61. MacKay RJ, Mallicote M, Hernandez JA, et al. A review of anhidrosis in horses. Equine Vet Educ 2015;27(4):192–9.
62. Jenkinson DM, Elder HY, Bovell DL. Equine sweating and anhidrosis Part 2: anhidrosis. Vet Dermatol 2007;18(1):2–11.
63. Jenkinson DM, Elder HY, Bovell DL. Equine sweating and anhidrosis Part 1 – equine sweating. Vet Dermatol 2006;17(6):361–92.
64. Shmalberg J, Xie H, Memon MA. Horses referred to a teaching hospital exclusively for acupuncture and herbs: a three-year retrospective analysis. J Acupunct Meridian Stud 2019;12(5):145–50.
65. Atria S, Carson E, Xie H, et al. Acupuncture and Chinese herbal medicine treatment of eighteen Florida horses with anhidrosis. Am J Tradit Chin Vet Med 2010; 5(2):25–35.

Rehabilitation
Proprioception, Incoordination, and Paresis

Melissa R. King, DVM, PhD

KEYWORDS

- Rehabilitation • Proprioception • Core strength • Therapeutic exercises

KEY POINTS

- The role of the muscle systems becomes even greater in the presence of injury or pathology
- Neuromuscular inefficiency as the result of regional pain and dysfunction must be addressed independently of the pathoanatomical diagnosis.
- Therapeutic exercise interventions are essential for the effective management of patients with pain and dysfunction.

INTRODUCTION

The ultimate goal of any rehabilitation program is to return an injured equine athlete to a fully functioning, pain-free state. To accomplish this, therapeutic programs must be customized to each individual addressing mechanisms to modulate pain, restore joint range of motion, enhance neuromotor control, improve muscle strength, and increase flexibility. An initial global evaluation assessing the horse's level of function and identification of primary and secondary structural and functional deficits aids the therapist in establishing a therapeutic program to address each problem. Subsequently, patient reevaluation occurs continually throughout the rehabilitation process resulting in changes based on progression and adaptation to the therapeutic protocol.

To date, there are significant gaps in the knowledge base regarding the phenomenon of pain and dysfunction in the horse. Regrettably, objective data evaluating integrative techniques and rehabilitative treatments for pain and dysfunction are scarce. Similarly, many of the therapies employed in rehabilitation programs often lack adequate scientific support. This does not necessarily mean that they are not effective, it simply means the optimal timing and usage of certain therapies is yet to be established. The focus of this article is to provide an overview of different integrative techniques available for global rehabilitation including the scientific basis, physiologic effects, and indications.

Colorado State University Veterinary Teaching Hospital, Equine Orthopaedic Research Center, 2250 Gillette Drive Fort Collins, CO 80523, USA
E-mail address: Melissa.king@colostate.edu

Vet Clin Equine 38 (2022) 557–568
https://doi.org/10.1016/j.cveq.2022.06.010
0749-0739/22/Published by Elsevier Inc.

Proprioceptive Facilitation Techniques in Horses

Mechanism of action

Recent human research has expanded our understanding of neuromuscular responses to joint pain.[1] Mechanoreceptors are characterized as sensory receptors within periarticular tissues that respond to changes in joint position and acceleration of movement, as well as playing an important role in regulating and maintaining neuromuscular control of joint stability.[2] Pain, inflammation, and joint effusion associated with osteoarthritis alter the normal sensory input from articular mechanoreceptors, which may result in decreased motor neuron excitability and reduced muscle activation.[3] A common outcome following experimentally induced knee effusion is the presence of significant quadriceps muscle inhibition.[4–7] A linear relationship exists between increased intra-articular pressure and the level of quadriceps inhibition.[4] Electromyography studies conducted on the quadriceps muscle of patients with knee osteoarthritis often indicate a decrease in muscle strength and altered muscle timing.[8] Typically there is a delay in the onset of quadriceps muscle activation, which results in the inability of the quadriceps to stabilize the joint and attenuate the loading forces properly during locomotion.[5] The increased joint instability further alters the distribution of weight-bearing forces across joint surfaces and increases the recruitment of adjacent muscles to aid in joint stability.[9] The resulting imbalances in paired agonist–antagonist muscle groups contribute to increased joint instability and altered limb biomechanics, which leads to progressive osteoarthritis and chronic maladaptive compensatory mechanisms.[10]

Similar results would be expected in horses, the presence of pain may lead to loss of function, diminished neuromotor control, decreased joint range of motion, and muscle atrophy. The application of various proprioceptive techniques is frequently used to increase joint range of motion, reestablish appropriate neuromuscular firing patterns, and improve the strength of targeted muscles that function to move and stabilize the joints.[11] The use of tactile stimulators applied around the hindlimb pastern showed a significantly higher hoof flight arc, with increased flexion of the fetlock, hock, and stifle joints (**Fig. 1**).[11] The use of this proprioceptive technique supports the facilitation of enhanced afferent input to indirectly produce and modulate a targeted efferent response for the purpose of reestablishing motor control and improving joint range of motion.

A multitude of other proprioceptive techniques are used from resistive bands and elastic therapeutic tape to ground poles and changes in ground surfaces. Resistance band training is successfully used in human physical therapy programs to improve core strength and stability.[12,13] Commonly referred to as a Theraband,[a] the two-piece equine elastic band system is thought to stimulate core abdominal muscles with the abdominal band and engage hindlimb musculature with the hindquarter band (**Fig. 2**). Its use in horses at a trot was recently investigated and found to reduce mediolateral and rotational movement throughout the thoracolumbar region.[14] Further studies investigating more long-term use and potential mechanistic pathways will help refine its use in the rehabilitation setting. Also pertinent to rehabilitation is the use of training lines. Pessoa training aids were shown to increase both lumbosacral angles and thoracolumbar dorsoventral excursion when used in horses being lunged at a jog.[15] Ground poles when arranged at various distances, heights and configurations can encourage an increase in the lateral thoracolumbar excursion (**Fig. 3**). Hill work and incorporating backing exercises into hill work can also be used to simultaneously

---

[a] Equiband, Equicore Concepts LLC Lansing, MI 48912.

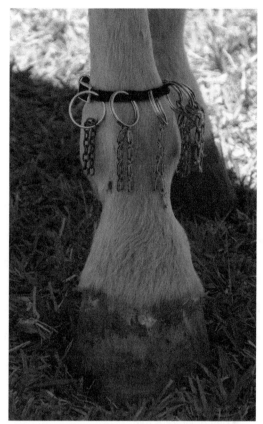

Fig. 1. Application of a tactile stimulator above the fetlock, used to provide a non-noxious sensory stimulus to encourage concentric flexor muscle activation to improve upper limb joint range of motion, neuromotor control, and muscle strength.

improve muscular strength and challenge proprioceptive acuity. Although further studies are needed to establish specific recommendations regarding use, initial biomechanical effects for targeted rehabilitation are encouraging.

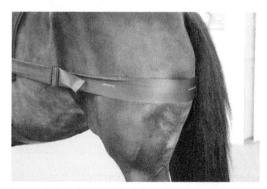

Fig. 2. Proprioceptive resistive bands placed around hindquarters and abdomen to encourage lumbosacral flexion, spinal stability, and increased hindlimb protraction.

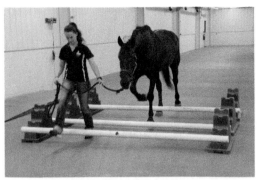

Fig. 3. Altered height position of caveletti poles used to alter proprioceptive input to encourage changes in limb range of motion, stride length, and neuromotor control.

Clinical application

- Ground poles can be used to increase both range of motion and stride length depending on height and distance of spacing.
  - Used in the early phases of rehabilitation during the hand walking sessions
  - Initially height is kept low and increased as the horse progresses through the program
  - Three to five poles in succession making two to five passes through the poles initially
  - As the horse progresses through the program the number of passes, the height, and position of the poles can be adjusted.
- Tactile stimulators can be applied to increase the range of motion during hand walking sessions
  - Protocol 2–3× a day daily for 5 min
  - Can lessen response (degree of flexion) by applying device to opposite limb initially
  - Habituate quickly to device within the same session thus apply for shorter periods of time multiple times a day
  - Owing to the degree of response (hyperflexion) caution starting too early in the rehabilitation process
- Resistance bands can be used to encourage lumbosacral flexion and increase hindlimb protraction when applied around hind quarters
  - Applied during hand walking sessions
    - Initially kept in place for 5 min during a single-hand walking session
    - Increase time at weekly increments until able to wear during a full hand walking session
    - Typically used once to twice a day
- Varied ground surfaces
  - Use during the hand walking sessions to promote motor control and core stability

Therapeutic Exercises

Mechanism of action

Physiotherapeutic exercises aimed at stimulating motor control, flexibility, and stability are regularly employed in human physical therapy programs. Specifically, the use of such exercises has been shown to reduce both pain and reinjury.[16–18] Pursuant to the equine patient, several core strengthening exercises and their role in activating deep epaxial musculature to subsequently improve postural motor control and alter thoracolumbar kinematics have been investigated.[18,19] Both baited and passive exercises offer opportunities to facilitate stretching during dynamic phases and strengthening during static phases of the exercise. Institution of dynamic mobilization exercises over a 3-month time period has been shown to increase both size and symmetry of the multifidus muscle as assessed through longitudinal ultrasonographic evaluation.[20,21] Blanket recommendations regarding prescription of exercises are not advised, individual patient prescription should be considered in the context of handler safety, specific rehabilitation goals, and patient ability to effectively complete the exercise.

Multiple human studies have shown that individuals with spinal pathology and back pain have reduced muscle cross-sectional area (CSA) leading to loss of function and impairments in postural control and proprioceptive acuity. Human athletes that incorporate core, balance exercises into their rehabilitation programs are significantly less likely to suffer reinjury during a 12-month period following injury, compared with those individuals with similar injuries that did not emphasize core strength (7% reinjury rate in the balance training group versus 29% reinjury rate in the control group).[22] Strengthening and improving proprioception and balance control following injury remain a central focus of human physical therapy programs, and although standardized investigations have yet to focus on equine applications, there are several mechanisms through which neuromotor control can be recruited. In a study evaluating postural sway in horses with experimentally induced carpal osteoarthritis, horses with improved postural stability following underwater treadmill exercise showed more symmetric limb loading than a control group.[23] This suggests that with improved postural stability, there is enhanced proprioception and neuromotor control critical to protecting the axial and appendicular skeleton. In addition, Ellis and colleagues[24] showed significant *musculus multifidus* hypertrophy together with improvements in postural stability in response to individualized rehabilitation programs involving a series of dynamic core strengthening and controlled rehabilitation exercises involving the use of balance proprioceptive pads (**Fig. 4**).

Passive Joint Range of Motion and Core Strengthening Exercises

Mechanism of action

Passive range of motion can be described as passively moving a joint or joints through the normal physiologic range of motion without muscular activity. The primary goals of

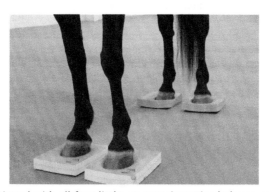

Fig. 4. Horse positioned with all four limbs on proprioceptive balance pads.

passive range of motion exercise are to prevent joint capsule fibrosis, maintain tissue mobility, improve vascular dynamics, allow for synovial fluid diffusion, and decrease pain. Passive range of motion exercise stretches those muscles whose action would actively move the joint, thus improving their contractile properties. In addition, the predominant clinical use of passive motion is to target peri-articular tissues in an attempt to prevent joint capsule fibrosis. Human clinical studies assessing passive range of motion exercises in patients following knee arthroplasty showed a significant improvement in range of motion that was still apparent after one year.[25,26] The improvement in range of motion can be supported by results in the rabbit models that demonstrate as healing occurs within the joint capsule, collagen fibers align randomly. This random, cross-linking pattern causes increased fibrosis and thickening of the capsule. Passive range of motion exercises is proposed to work at a cellular level by decreasing the random alignment of the collagen fibers through stimulation of physiologic motion enhancing parallel fiber orientation.[27]

Clinical Application

Passive flexion/extension exercises are typically conducted once to twice a day with two sets of 30–50 cycles per joint of interest. As the horse progresses gradually, increase either the number of sets or the number of reps. Caution: only increase one portion at a time; do not increase both the number of sets and the number of reps at the same time. If chronic capsulitis is present it may help to heat the tissues first.

Core strengthening exercises have been recommended to reduce stiffness, enhance soft-tissue mobilization, increase muscle activation, lengthen the musculotendinous unit, decrease pain, and improve performance. A recent imaging study assessed the CSA of the thoracolumbar multifidi muscles in horses with clinical signs of back pain.[20] Those horses with evidence of osseous pathologic changes showed a measurable asymmetry in the multifidus muscle CSA at the level of the pathology.[20] In a follow-up study, regular performance of dynamic mobilization exercises was shown to increase *multifidus* muscle CSA from T10 to L5.[21] Eight clinically sound horses performed five repetitions of mobilization exercises 5 days per week, over a three-month period. The exercises consisted of three cervical flexion positions, one cervical extension position, and three lateral bending positions to the left and right sides. The results of the study showed that the CSA of the thoracolumbar multifidi muscles increased in size in response to the mobilization exercises.[21] The increase in multifidus muscle development following dynamic mobilization is a promising rehabilitative technique for horses in which this muscle has atrophied due to back pain.

The effect of core abdominal muscle rehabilitation exercises on return to training and performance in horses after colic surgery showed that 82% of horses in the core exercise group improved their level of performance beyond their level before surgery, versus only 8% in the none core exercise group.[28] Those horses enrolled in the treatment group began a set of core exercises 30 days post-colic surgery, conducting the sets once daily, 5 days a week for four weeks.[28] All horses were followed out for one year.[28] The initiation of core abdominal exercises following colic surgery may have facilitated faster convalescence and improved performance.

Clinical Application

Cervical spinal range of motion exercises is achieved when the horse follows a controlled movement pattern that recruits both the dynamic mobilizing muscles and the deep stabilizing muscles used to round or bend the neck.[19] The horse is taught to follow a controlled movement pattern using bait, such as a piece of carrot, through a specific movement pattern that involves rounding and/or lateral bending of the neck while stabilizing the back and limbs to maintain balance.[21] A series of dynamic mobilization exercises are often used to induce flexion, extension, and lateral bending throughout the cervical spine to reduce stiffness and improve range of motion through portions of the thoracolumbar region as well. These baited, active-assisted range of motion exercises can be divided into three flexed positions: (1) chin to chest targets flexion of the upper cervical spine, (2) chin between carpi increases flexion of mid-to-caudal cervical spine, and (3) chin between fetlock increases flexion of mid-to-caudal cervical spine and activation of the rectus abdominus to contract and lift the back.[21] When asking the horse to bend laterally into three positions using a baited, active assisted range of motion exercise, the chin to girth showed the greatest degree of lateral flexion occurring at C1.[21] Bending chin to hip and chin to tarsus both increased lateral bending in the caudal cervical spine with the majority of lateral flexion occurring at C6-T1 and induced lateral bending within the thoracolumbar region as well. The optimal time to perform dynamic mobilization is immediately before exercise each day to pre-activate the postural control muscles. The horse is encouraged to hold the position for several seconds and after each exercise allow the muscles to relax for several seconds. Perform three to five repetitions of each exercise per day (3–4 days a week) and, for the lateral bending exercises, do an equal number of repetitions to the left and right sides.[21]

Elastic Therapeutic Tape

Mechanism of action
Elastic therapeutic tape is an adhesive product designed for use in treating sports injuries and a variety of other musculoskeletal disorders in humans. Manufacturers claim that elastic therapeutic tape supports injured muscles and joints and helps to relieve pain and edema by lifting the skin and allowing improved blood and lymph flow.[29] A review of the current human literature suggests that elastic therapeutic tape may have a small beneficial role in improving cutaneous proprioception, strength, and joint range of motion, but further studies are needed to confirm these findings.[29] Studies have shown effects on underlying muscle activity, but it is unclear whether these changes are beneficial or harmful in the management and prevention of specific human sports injuries. Equine certification courses have been initiated; however, the current level of evidence for use in treating musculoskeletal disorders is largely anecdotal, but promising results have been appreciated with preliminary investigations incorporating the use of pressure algometry pre- and post-application (King, unpublished data, 2021). Elastic therapeutic taping is used clinically most often to promote changes in motion and limb function.

Clinical application
Application of elastic therapeutic tape is often applied for the management of focal swelling and edema, to reduce myofascial restriction and for the purposes of muscle activation (**Fig. 5**). The hair will need to be clean with no dirt or debris and no-fly spray or coat conditioners applied. The tape will typically stay in place for 3–5 days at which point reassessment should take place to determine if reapplication is necessary.

Whole-Body Vibration

Whole-body vibration therapy (WBV) involves the application of low frequency, low-amplitude mechanical stimulation for therapeutic purposes. The response of the equine musculoskeletal tissues to vibration stimuli is determined by the frequency, direction (vertical versus oscillatory), magnitude (displacement and acceleration), and the duration of therapy. As a result of the large number of vibration factor interactions

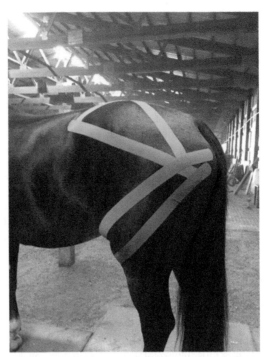

Fig. 5. Showing the application of elastic therapeutic tape post-stifle surgery to encourage proprioceptive input to the stifle extensors and encourage functional release of the stifle.

WBV guidelines for enhancing musculoskeletal tissue responses have not been determined in the horse. Multiple studies conducted in rodent and ovine models of fracture repair demonstrate the diversified vibration protocols including variations in frequency, magnitude, and duration. Both closed and open fracture repair models in rodents demonstrate that vertical vibration at a frequency of 45 Hz negatively impairs fracture healing while vibration frequencies of 35 and 50 Hz enhance fracture healing. In contrast, horizontal oscillatory vibration therapy regardless of frequency demonstrates no positive or negative effects on fracture healing in rodent models.[30] Peripheral blood flow and tissue oxygenation in people have been shown to be positively influenced by WBV.[31] The mechanical oscillations transferred from the vibration plate to elderly individuals have improved postural control and thus have reduced the risk of falling within the elderly population.[22,32] Furthermore, there is modest evidence that supports the use of vibration therapy to reduce pain perception in osteoarthritic individuals.[33,34] Lastly, there is an emerging profile for the application of vibration therapy as an exercise modality for people. Vibration training for human athletes appears to have a rapid and energy sparring warm-up effect and has shown increases in jump height and muscle power.[35,36]

A translational comparison within the human literature to the horse becomes very difficult as a number of different WBV platforms are commercially available. Anecdotally, WBV has been applied to horses with various claims of effectiveness. Acute hematologic and clinical effects of horses undergoing alternating horizontal and vertical vibration therapy have been recently described, noting no adverse effects following vibration sessions exposed to a frequency of 15–21 Hz.[37] Within the rehabilitative setting, there has been recent interest in the effects of prolonged vibration therapy on the CSA and symmetry of the multifidus muscle. A significant increase in multifidus muscle cross-sectional size and symmetry was found following 60 days of twice daily, 30 min, 40 Hz vertical WBV sessions.[38] Known for its role in spinal stabilization and postural muscle acuity, the development of the multifidus muscle is thought to have potential as an osteoarthritis deterrent. Only one study has been conducted on the horse evaluating the effects of vibration therapy on bone density in stalled patients. Twelve horses were confined to stalls for 60 days with half the group exercised daily on a mechanical walker and the others underwent vertical WBV therapy at 50 Hz for 45 min, 5 days a week.[39] WBV therapy in stalled horses maintained the same bone mineral content to that of horses that received daily light exercise and therefore should be considered for horses restricted to stall rest only.[39] However, to date no direct comparison studies on vibration direction in the horse have been conducted.

Clinical application
Whole-body exercise appears to be a safe method for rehabilitation in the horse, but additional studies are needed to assess efficacy in equine patients for stimulating bone metabolism, soft-tissue healing, proprioceptive awareness, and motor control mechanisms responsible for joint stability and movement patterns. Manufacturer recommendations for treatment protocols typically involve twice-daily 30-min treatment sessions at varied frequencies. Still largely unknown to the equine community is the evidence-based support for the appropriately combined settings of frequency, direction (vertical versus oscillatory), magnitude (displacement and acceleration), and the duration of therapy for a specific musculoskeletal injury.

SUMMARY

Developing a successful rehabilitation protocol involves first reaching an accurate diagnosis followed by establishing clearly defined rehabilitation goals. Although the general goals of rehabilitation are usually similar—to first decrease pain and inflammation while preventing further injury and then to restore normal function by restoring proprioception, flexibility, strength, and endurance—there is often significant variation in rehabilitation protocols. For example, the protocol may vary based on the duration, type, and severity of the injury, the goals and finances of the owner, available rehabilitation equipment and resources, and the intended use of the horse.

CLINICS CARE POINTS

- In human athletes poor core stability increases risk of injury. Similar results would be expected in our equine athletes.
- Rehabilitative strategies have demonstrated a significant strong correlation between *musculus multifidus* cross-sectional area (CSA) and postural stability in lame horses undergoing a rehabilitation program. These findings suggest that a rehabilitation program that includes core strengthening helps improve spinal muscle characteristics and postural stability.
- Move beyond just addressing the pathoanatomical diagnosis, conduct a global examine to determine the functional impairments and additional co-morbidities that have developed as a result of the primary injury.

DISCLOSURE

The author has nothing to disclose.

REFERENCES

1. Templeton MS, Booth DL, O'Kelly WD. Effects of aquatic therapy on joint flexibility and functional ability in subjects with rheumatic disease. J Orthop Sports Phys Ther 1996;23:376–81.
2. Hurley MV. The effects of joint damage on muscle function, proprioception and rehabilitation. Man Ther 1997;2:11–7.
3. Johansson H, Sjolander P, Sojka P. A sensory role for the cruciate ligaments. Clin Orthop 1991;268:161–78.
4. Hopkins J, Ingersoll C, Edwards J, et al. Changes in soleus motor neuron pool excitability after artificial knee joint effusion. Arch Phys Med Rehabil 2000;81: 1199–203.
5. Hopkins J, Ingersoll C, Krause B, et al. Effect of knee joint effusion on quadriceps and soleus motor neuron pool excitability. Med Sports Sci Sports Exerc 2001;33: 123–6.
6. Iles J, Stokes M, Young A. Reflex actions of knee joint afferents during contraction of the human quadriceps. Clin Physiol 1990;10:489–500.
7. Palmieri R, Tom J, Edwards J, et al. Arthrogenic muscle response induced by an experimental knee joint effusion is mediated by pre- and post-synaptic spinal mechanisms. J Electromyogr Kinesiol 2004;14:631–40.
8. Dixon J, Howe T. Quadriceps force generation in patients with osteoarthritis of the knee and asymptomatic participants during patellar tendon reflex reactions: an exploratory cross-sectional study. BMC Musculoskelet Disord 2005; 6:1–6.
9. Shultz SJ, Carcia CR, Perrin DH. Knee joint laxity affects muscle activation patterns in the healthy knee. J Electromyogr Kinesiol 2004;14:475–83.
10. Wu S-H, Chu N-K, Liu Y-C, et al. Relationship between the EMG ratio of muscle activation and bony structure in osteoarthritic knee patients with and without patellar malalignment. J Rehabil Med 2008;40:381–6.
11. Clayton HM, White AD, Kaiser LJ, et al. Hindlimb response to tactile stimulation of the pastern and coronet. Equine Vet J 2010;42:227–33.
12. Kell RT, Asmundson GJG. A comparison of two forms of periodized exercise rehabilitation programs in the management of chronic nonspecific low-back pain. J Strength Cond Res 2009;23:513–23.
13. Macedo LG, Maher CG, Latimer J, et al. Motor control exercise for persistent, nonspecific low back pain: a systematic review. Phys Ther 2009; 89:9–25.
14. Pfau T, Simons V, Rombach N, et al. Effect of a 4-week elastic resistance band training regimen on back kinematics in horses trotting in-hand and on the lunge. Equive Vet J 2017;49:829–35.
15. Walker VA, Dyson SJ, Murray RC. Effect of a Pessoa training aid on temporal, linear and angular variables of the working trot. Vet J 2013;198:404–41.
16. Hides JA, Jull GA, Richardson CA. Long-term effects of specific stabilizing exercises for first-episode low back pain. Spine 2001;26:E243–8.
17. O'Sullivan PB, Phyty GD, Tworney LT, et al. Evaluation of Specific Stabilizing Exercise in the Treatment of Chronic Low Back Pain With Radiologic Diagnosis of Spondylolysis or Spondylolisthesis. Spine 1997;22(24):2959–67.
18. Kavcic N, Grenier S, McGill SM. Determining the Stabilizing Role of Individual Torso Muscles During Rehabilitation Exercises. Spine 2004;29(11):1254–65.

19. Clayton HM, Kaiser LJ, Lavagnino M, et al. Dynamic mobilizations in cervical flexion: Effects on intervertebral angulations. Equine Vet J 2010;42(Suppl s38): 688–94.
20. Stubbs NC, Riggs CM, Hodges PW, et al. Osseous spinal pathology and epaxial muscle ultrasonography in Thoroughbred racehorses. Equine Vet J 2010;42: 654–61.
21. Stubbs NC, Kaiser LJ, Hauptman J, et al. Dynamic mobilisation exercises increase cross-sectional area of musculus multifidus. Equine Vet J 2011;43(5): 522–9.
22. Holme E, Magnusson SP, Becher K, et al. The effect of supervised rehabilitation on strength, postural sway, position sense and re-injury risk after acute ankle sprain. Scand J Med Sci Sports 1999;9:104–9.
23. King MR, Haussler KK, Kawcak CE, et al. Effect of underwater treadmill exercise on postural sway in horses with experimentally induced carpal joint osteoarthritis. Am J Vet Res 2013;74(7):971–82.
24. Ellis KL, King MR. Relationship between postural stability and paraspinal muscle adaptation in lame horses undergoing rehabilitation. J Equine Vet Sci 2020. https://doi.org/10.1016/j.evs.2020.103108.
25. Salter R, Hamilton H, Wedge J, et al. Clinical application of basic research on continuous passive motion for disorders and injuries of synovial joints: A preliminary report of a feasibility study. J Orthop Res 1984;1:325–42.
26. Salter S, Simmond D, Malcom B, et al. The biological effect of continuous passive motion of the healing of full - thickness defects in articular cartilage. J Bone Joint Surg 1980;62:1232–51.
27. Ferretti M, Srinivasan A, Deschner J, et al. Anti-inflammatory effects of continuous passive motion on meniscal fibrocartilage. J Orthop Res 2005;23:1165–71.
28. Holcombe SJ, Shearer TR, Valberg SJ. The effect of core abdominal muscle rehabilitation exercises on return to training and performance in horses after colic surgery. J Equine Vet Sci 2019;75:14–8.
29. Williams S, Whatman C, Hume PA, et al. Kinesio taping in treatment and prevention of sports injuries: a meta-analysis of the evidence for its effectiveness. Sports Med 2011;42:153–64.
30. Wang J, Leung KS, Chow SKH, et al. The effect of whole body vibration on fracture healing – A systematic review. Eurp Cells Mater 2017;34:108–27.
31. Games KE, Sefton JM, Wilson AE. Whole-body vibration and blood flow and muscle oxygenation: a meta-analysis. J Athl Train 2015;50:542–9.
32. Verschueren S, Roelants M, Delecluse C, et al. Effect of 6-month whole body vibration training on hip density, muscle strength, and postural control in postmenopausal women: a randomized controlled pilot study. J Bone Miner Res 2004;19:352–9.
33. Park YG, Kwon BS, Park J-W, et al. Therapeutic effect of whole body vibration on chronic knee osteoarthritis. Ann Rehabil Med 2013;37(4):505–15.
34. Perraton L, Machotka Z, Kumar S. Whole-body vibration to treat low back pain: fact or fad? Physiother Can 2011;63(1):88–93.
35. Bagheri J, Van den berg-emons R, Pel J, et al. Acute effects of whole-body vibration on jump force and jump rate of force development: a comparative study of different devices. J Strength Cond Res 2012;26:691–6.
36. Rehn B, Lidstrom J, Skoglund J, et al. Effects of leg muscular performance from whole-body vibration exercise: a systematic review. Scand J Med Sci Sports 2007;17:2–11.

37. Carstanjen B, Balali M, Gajewski Z, et al. Short-term whole body vibration exercise in adult healthy horses. Pol J Vet Sci 2013;16(2):403–5.
38. Halsberghe BT, Gordon-Ross P, Peterson R. Whole body vibration affects the cross-sectional area and symmetry of the m. multifidus of the thoracolumbar spine in the horse. Eq Vet E 2017;29(9):493–9.
39. Hulak ES, Spooner HS, Haffner JC. Influence of whole-body vibration on bone density in the stalled horse. J Eq Vet Sc 2015;35(5):393.

Therapeutic Exercises for Equine Sacroiliac Joint Pain and Dysfunction

Lesley Goff, PhD, MAnimSt(AnimPhysio), MAppSc(ExSpSc), GDipAppSc(ManipPhysio), BAppSc(Physio)

KEYWORDS

- Sacroiliac joint • Therapeutic exercise • Posture • Dynamic • Hypomobility
- Joint motion • Pain

KEY POINTS

- There are no preset rules for therapeutic exercise prescription.
- Each horse should be assessed individually for their specific functional impairments.
- Prescription of the exercise program should include consideration of issues related to functional instability versus the articular hypomobility.
- When introducing a therapeutic exercise or modality, the effect of the exercise or modality should be reassessed before progressing with further treatment.

Video content accompanies this article at http://www.vetequine.theclinics. com.

INTRODUCTION

Rehabilitation is defined as restoration to a prior level of function. Rehabilitation of the sacroiliac joint can be challenging, as the presence of pain and dysfunction is varied and onset is often insidious. Therapeutic exercise involves the prescription of specified movements to help reduce pain and impairments and to restore musculoskeletal function. The role of therapeutic exercise in the rehabilitation of sacroiliac joint pain and dysfunction in horses has not been well established. The goal is to provide the reader with some contemporary knowledge and evidence where possible, so that clinical reasoning can be used to formulate an exercise plan that is specific to the clinical presentation.

FUNCTIONAL ANATOMY

To understand the function of the sacroiliac joint, it is useful to briefly review the anatomy. The sacroiliac joint is located within the pelvis of the horse, between the ilium

School of Veterinary Science, University of Queensland, Active Animal Physiotherapy and Hip Sport Spine Physiotherapy, PO Box 277, Highfields, QLD 4350, Australia
E-mail address: lesley@animalphysio.com.au

Vet Clin Equine 38 (2022) 569–584
https://doi.org/10.1016/j.cveq.2022.07.002
0749-0739/22/© 2022 Elsevier Inc. All rights reserved.

dorsally and the sacrum ventrally. The sacral articular surface of the sacroiliac joint is covered in hyaline cartilage, a tissue designed to take compressive load. Hyaline cartilage also provides a very low coefficient of friction, which facilitates smooth translatory joint surface motion. The ilial articular surface is covered in fibrocartilage, which can resist high degrees of tension as well as compression.[1] Movements at the sacroiliac joint are complex and not well understood; although, we do know that the magnitude of relative movement between the ilium and sacrum is small.[2,3] However, we do not know of the magnitude of compression and translation at the joint surface that occurs during loading and locomotion.

The sacroiliac ligaments include an interosseus ligament, a thin ventral ligament, the broad sacrosciatic ligament, which is a sheet-like structure providing attachment for some muscles of the pelvis, and the dorsal sacroiliac ligament, which changes in cross-sectional area with movement of the ilium relative to the sacrum.[3] Each ligament functions to limit motion between the sacrum and pelvis. Because of the relationship with the overlying musculature, the lateral portion of the dorsal sacroiliac ligament and the broad sacrosciatic ligament may function in assisting the transfer of propulsive forces from the hind limb musculature, which has long been considered a role of the sacroiliac joint in general.[4] In human studies it has been established that coordination of muscle groups of the lumbopelvic region can affect stability at the sacroiliac joint[5]; this may also be the case in the horse. Restoration of the transfer of propulsive forces and local muscle coordination is required for full rehabilitation of sacroiliac pain and dysfunction. Therefore, the combination of rest and pain management is often not sufficient for rehabilitation of the equine sacroiliac joint. In fact, rest may be detrimental to recovery. To attain the optimal outcome in equine sacroiliac joint rehabilitation, the specific prescription of rehabilitative exercise is paramount, as the rehabilitation plan and the type of therapeutic exercises depend on the type and location of sacroiliac pain and dysfunction that is present.

SACROILIAC PAIN AND DYSFUNCTION

There are 2 possible clinical presentations of sacroiliac pain and dysfunction in horses.[6] One occurs in performance horses in work that present with nonspecific clinical signs of poor hind limb impulsion, thoracolumbar and lumbosacral stiffness, and a tendency to be above the bit, which are resolved by local anesthesia of the sacroiliac joint region.[7] The specific pathologic changes associated with this type of sacroiliac joint dysfunction are not well understood. Only 43% of horses with a positive response to local anesthetic had abnormal radioactive uptake with scintigraphy and only 32% of horses that underwent per rectum ultrasonographic examination had documented sacroiliac joint abnormalities. The described response to local anesthetic injection may be associated with pain in periarticular structures such as that occurs in humans,[8] rather than more specific osteoarthritic changes associated with the sacroiliac joint itself. Perhaps these clinical presentations represent sacroiliac joint ligament or adjacent muscle injury or a functional joint instability related to altered biomechanics and neuromotor control.[9] The positive response of some horses to local anesthesia could also indicate the presence of inflammation (desmitis), as the sacroiliac ligaments are known to be pain-producing structures in humans.[10]

The other form of sacroiliac joint dysfunction has been reported as being associated with chronic sacroiliac joint pathology.[11] In these cases, there may be more marked gait abnormalities and the presence of more noticeable muscle and bony asymmetry. These horses show little improvement to regional analgesia.[11] Indeed, one horse that is reported in Barstow and Dyson (2015)[9] had clinical signs typical of sacroiliac joint region pain and did not respond to local analgesia, but at postmortem examination it had extensive degenerative changes of the sacroiliac joints. These 2 variations of sacroiliac joint dysfunction may represent the opposing ends of the spectrum in a continuum of sacroiliac joint dysfunction (**Fig. 1**), which require different rehabilitation approaches.

JOINT MOTION

When prescribing therapeutic exercises for sacroiliac joint pain and dysfunction, it is useful to understand the concepts of joint neutral zone, muscle systems, and the effects of altered joint loading.

NEUTRAL ZONE

The neutral zone is defined as the portion of the physiologic joint range of motion, measured from a neutral joint position, where there is minimal internal resistance.[12] It is a clinically important measure of spinal stability function that can be applied to the sacroiliac joint. Panjabi (1992)[12] described the concept of the neutral zone and the nonlinear behavior of joints subjected to load (**Fig. 2**). Joints have increased flexibility and are more mobile at low loads and stiffen as joint loading increases.

Increases and decreases in the neutral zone are due to multiple factors.[13,14] The neutral zone is theorized to be reduced due to the presence of muscle hypertonicity or osteophytes, which may physically stabilize joint motion.[15] The neutral zone may increase at certain stages of joint degeneration, ligamentous injury, or with muscular weakness or incoordination. An increase in the neutral zone combined with reduced motor control may be termed a functional instability. The neutral zone may be modified by using a rehabilitative motor control approach, which consists of improved coordination of stabilizing and global musculature, which is outlined later.

MUSCLE SYSTEMS

There are no muscles that have a direct or isolated effect on the sacroiliac joint; therefore, the focus in rehabilitation is to affect the multisegmented muscles that traverse the sacroiliac joint and form attachments on the distant lumbar vertebrae, pelvis, or proximal femur. Two groups of muscles may be considered related to sacroiliac joint function[1]: stabilizing muscles, which contribute to joint stiffness, reduce the neutral zone, and are characterized by an early onset of activation in response to perturbation,[16] and[2] global muscles, which include muscles of powerful or fast movement required for locomotion.[9] Deep, segmental muscles mainly contribute to spinal stability, whereas global muscles have more of a role of being prime movers, are more superficial, and do

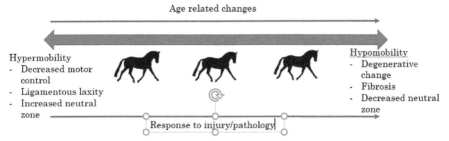

Fig. 1. The proposed continuum of equine sacroiliac joint dysfunction.

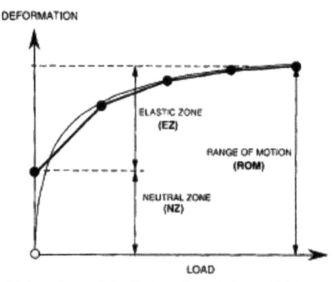

Fig. 2. A load-deformation graph that illustrates the neutral zone of joint movement that is characterized by joint range of motion with minimal or no load. *Adapted from* Panjabi (1992).[12]

not provide segmental stability[17]; although, some muscles have dual roles. The muscle's ability to perform a role is related to the muscle fiber type—slow twitch (type I) and fast twitch, highly oxidative (type IIA/2A) and fast twitch, low oxidative (type IIB/2X) identified on histochemistry and characterized by the myosin chain isoforms.[9] Muscle fiber types dictate the power produced and the resistance to fatigue.

The multifidus muscle in the thoracolumbar region is described as having the action of extending, laterally bending, and axially rotating vertebrae but is thought to have a dual role of stabilizing and locomotion due to the proportion of fast twitch fibers (50%).[9] Two muscles that arise from the sacrum and attach to the caudal vertebrae include the sacrocaudalis dorsalis medialis and sacrocaudalis dorsalis lateralis, which are considered an extension of the multifidus muscle into the sacral and caudal regions. These muscles have a very low proportion of fast twitch fibers (16%), so they may have a dual role of moving the tail, as well as providing sacrocaudal stabilization. The psoas minor muscle, which originates from the caudal thoracic and lumbar regions and attaches to the brim of the pelvis, has a high proportion of type I muscle fibers that provide stabilization to the lumbopelvic region and contribute to proprioception.[9]

The longissimus and middle gluteal muscles in horses have high percentages of fast twitch fibers (85%–90%), which suggests a dynamic function needed for locomotion. The lumbar portion of the iliocostalis and proximal portion of the biceps femoris muscles, which crosses the sacroiliac joint and attaches to the sacrum, both have slightly less proportion of fast twitch fibers. The psoas major and sacrocaudalis dorsalis lateralis muscles are thought to have a dual role of stabilization and locomotion.[9]

Understanding fiber type distribution in such a clinically important area can help direct clinicians in devising a therapeutic exercise program for horses with sacroiliac joint dysfunction. If we consider the continuum of sacroiliac joint dysfunction, it will help us to decide on whether the therapeutic exercise program should focus on the stabilizing muscles that provide joint stability and neuromotor control or the global muscles that contribute to strength and locomotor movements. A functionally designed therapeutic exercise program will incorporate muscles from both systems in appropriate proportions, as muscles from the 2 systems rarely work in isolation; this may involve breaking down the prescribed motor task into individual components and to consider how muscles function with respect to concentric and eccentric contractions.[9]

ALTERED JOINT LOADING

Articular cartilage health is based on nutrition supplied via intermittent loading and the related circulation of synovial fluid.[18,19] Animal studies have shown that unloading of a joint, or decrease in mechanical stimuli, combined with poor muscular control and weakness may predispose to articular cartilage atrophy and degeneration.[19] Altered weight bearing or abnormal load transfer through the sacroiliac joint may result from direct trauma to the lumbopelvic region or proximal hind limb due to a fall or microtrauma secondary to hind limb lameness or chronic repetitive use injuries. Direct trauma may cause disruption to the sacroiliac joint surface (**Fig. 3**) or sacroiliac ligament injury, laxity, or rupture.[14] Compromise of neuromotor control of muscles acting on the sacroiliac joint region[14] may be due to primary muscle injury, altered timing or activation of muscle, reflex pain inhibition, or hind limb lameness, which can alter the transmission of both tensioning and compressive forces through the sacroiliac articular surfaces; this may result in a functional instability or increased neutral zone that could contribute to early degenerative changes within the sacroiliac joint.

Goff and colleagues (2014)[20] and Haussler and colleagues (1999)[21] examined sacroiliac joints from 36 and 37 Thoroughbred racehorses, respectively and observed similar degenerative changes that included but were not limited to joint margin and intraarticular osteophytes and areas of subchondral bony reactivity. These studies are consistent with the findings of Jeffcott (1985)[11] and highlight the fact that articular changes commonly associated with aging and joint injury can occur in relatively young horses that are actively competing.

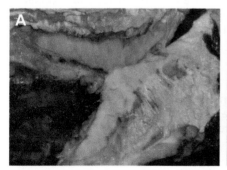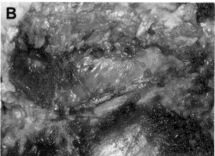

Fig. 3. (*A, B*) Photographs of gross necropsy specimens from the right (*A*) and left (*B*) sacroiliac joints of a 3-year-old filly that fell on left side of the pelvis and was subsequently euthanized. The right ilial and sacral articular surfaces (*A*) are clearly defined and are considered normal with minimal pathologic changes. In comparison, the left articular surfaces (*B*) are ill defined due to the surrounding tissue discolored with hemorrhage.

CLINICAL SIGNS

In summary, horses suspected to have sacroiliac joint dysfunction, particularly those with a functional instability, may or may not have positive findings on scintigraphic or transrectal ultrasonographic examination. The primary clinical signs may be less specific and related to poor performance and subtle observable or palpatory signs. These signs may include the following:

- Altered or unusual gait; hind limb plaiting at the trot; bunny hopping at the canter due to reduced ability to load and transmit forces through the sacroiliac joint[7]
- Difficulty performing static unilateral weight bearing on a hind limb, especially with perturbation due to reduced ability of the sacroiliac ligaments to support the sacroiliac joint and altered motor control[7]
- Reduced mobility in the thoracolumbar region due to muscle hypertonicity and guarding and observed trunk stiffness during exercise[5]
- Asymmetry of the pelvic musculature or overt pelvic muscle atrophy, which may be neurogenic or due to reduced weight bearing
- Pelvic bony landmark asymmetry due to postural alterations or due to a mechanical trauma to the pelvic region, such as a fall
- Tenderness over the dorsal sacroiliac ligament and middle gluteal muscle due to hypertonicity in the longissimus and gluteal musculature with subfailure of supporting ligamentous structures[12]
- Poor hind limb impulsion[3,7]

Other clinical signs such as poor contact with the bit, canter quality worse than movements at the trot, and bucking or kicking out with a hind limb during canter are reported to be worse during ridden work than during lunging.[7] These signs suggest an interrelationship between pain, increased neutral zone related to laxity in the passive stabilizing structures (ligaments), and alterations in the active stabilizing structures, which include the surrounding musculature and the neural pathways that contribute to motor control.[9]

PAIN LOCALIZATION AND EXERCISE

The use of local diagnostic anesthesia is often required to allow horses to move with less pain during exercise. In a study of 296 horses with sacroiliac regional pain, a high percentage showed an improvement in clinical signs during ridden exercise after periarticular local anesthesia.[7] The horses were walked for 15 minutes after local anesthesia and then either lunged or ridden with immediate changes in their gait noted. However, the clinical signs associated with sacroiliac joint dysfunction often develop over time and the onset is insidious.

REHABILITATION CONSIDERATIONS

Evidence from human studies suggest that prescribed therapeutic exercises for sacroiliac joint pain is beneficial in both the short and longer term.[22,23] Development of a therapeutic exercise program for sacroiliac joint pain and dysfunction needs to include the following considerations:

- Severity and distribution of pain
- Functional instability (hypermobility) of the sacroiliac joint
- Stiffness (hypomobility) of the sacroiliac joint or region

To aid in the clinical diagnosis, a functional assessment, detailed palpation of the muscles and adjacent soft tissues, and motion palpation of the quality and quantity of movements of the ilium, sacrum, and the lumbosacral junction are required. It is beyond the scope of this article to address the specific details of these examination procedures.

Rehabilitation of Sacroiliac Joint Instability

Goals for managing sacroiliac joint instability
- Manage pain
- Restore optimal articular motion
- Implement specific exercises to target the observed functional deficits
  - Type of exercise
  - Dosage—intensity, duration, frequency
  - Number of repetitions
  - Speed and timing of repetitions
  - When to perform exercises
- Activation of stabilization muscles
- Specific muscle activation
- Functional muscle activation
- Training aids
- Physical modalities
- Interpreting outcomes

Manage Pain

Pain management is paramount and often addressed as the first step in a rehabilitation program. Pain is primarily addressed through medical management by using nonsteroidal antiinflammatory drugs or periarticular infiltration of corticosteroids around the sacroiliac joint. Alternatively, or in conjunction with medical management, gentle manual therapy and dry needling are known to have pain-modulating neurophysiological effects via descending pain inhibition, pain gate mechanisms, and reflex muscle relaxation.[24] Electrotherapeutic agents such as transcutaneous electrical nerve stimulation or extracorporeal shockwave therapy have purported effects on axial skeleton pain, particularly for periarticular structures. Prescribing low-load, comfortable exercise in hand or at slow speeds is considered in acute phases of injury. Stall confinement or forced rest is contraindicated.

Restore Optimal Articular Motion

Even in horses with functional sacroiliac joint instability, it is useful to restore an optimal quality of sacroiliac joint and lumbosacral joint motion before instituting therapeutic exercises. Normalized joint motion may allow the musculature to work at optimal length-tension[25] and can be achieved via passive and active mobilization and manipulation. A skilled manual therapist is required to perform these techniques.

Implement Specific Exercises to Target the Observed Functional Deficits

The following section provides an overview and some examples of therapeutic exercises for sacroiliac joint dysfunction. The goal of therapeutic exercise prescription is to use the appropriate activity required to enhance motor control within an individual patient.

Dosage of Exercises

Contemporary views on dosages of exercise are based on the concepts that the physiologic response to physical interventions is individual and depends on various influencing factors.[26] Individualization is an emerging approach to exercise prescription with the aims of

- Maximizing the efficiency of an intervention by considering the specific needs of an equine athlete
- Considering the specific requirements of rehabilitation based on the type and severity of injury or dysfunction

Dosage of the prescribed exercises depends on

- The specific activity that we wish to rehabilitate
- Muscle type and fatiguability
- Owner and trainer abilities

It is key that the dosage is specific to the desired function and capability of the horse.[9]

Number of Repetitions

As it is impractical to use surface electromyography in the clinical setting, observation of the quality of the muscle activation and postural changes associated with the onset of fatigue may be used to determine the number of repetitions to deliver within a rehabilitation setting.[27]

Speed and Timing of Repetitions

The speed and timing of repetitions can be customized to reflect the desired activity. For example, in encouraging a horse to activate a muscle of hind limb propulsion required for a walking pace, the duration of delivery of the exercise that produces muscle activation should emulate the duration of that horse's stance phase of gait. The speed and timing will differ between horse size and breed. In the prescription of more complex therapeutic exercises, the exercise should be specific to the requirements of the skill or gait to deliver the optimal dosage of speed and timing. An example of a more complex exercise would be preparing or retraining the dressage horse for passage or piaffe, where ridden exercise and well-timed cues are required for the activity. The speed of the ridden exercise is varied, as the rider induces a reduction in stride length and speed as the horse transitions from a trot on a straight line to a small 10-m circle.

When to Perform Exercises

An ideal time to perform stabilizing muscle exercises is before or early in a sequence of in-hand, lunged, or ridden work. Newell and Rosenbloom (1982) state that the "most and fastest learning, and thus greatest improvement in performance, happens at the beginning of the practice period."[9] It is suggested that for optimal performance outcomes, practice of a given technique or exercise may require at least the same amount, or more time for rest than practice, during a training session.[9] This point is useful to consider not just in training muscles of stabilization but for prescribing other forms of therapeutic exercise.

Activation of Muscles of Stabilization

Core stability is a term originating from human rehabilitation that includes the lumbo-pelvic-hip complex and refers to the 3-dimensional muscular compartment formed by the abdominal muscles (anterior), diaphragm (dorsal), paraspinal and gluteal (posterior), and pelvic floor and hip muscles (ventral).[28,29] The term "core stability" is also used routinely in equine rehabilitation; however, we cannot directly extrapolate the role of the core stabilizing musculature from the bipedal to quadrupedal setting. It is likely that some of the muscles of spinal stabilization in humans may also serve a similar role in horses, which include the multifidus muscle and its caudal extension that forms the dorsal sacrocaudalis medialis and lateralis muscles.[30]

Neuromuscular (motor) control involves coordinated contraction (ie, timing, amplitudes) of both deep and superficial muscles[28]; therefore, the epaxial, intercostal, abdominal, and pelvic muscles are intricately interrelated in maintaining vertebral column equilibrium or stability. Stabilization of the sacroiliac joint and lumbosacral region are provided by the following muscles[30]:

- Dorsal sacrocaudalis medialis and lateralis
- Multifidus
- Psoas minor
- Abdominal muscles
- Diaphragm

These muscles provide core stability during locomotion and more advanced sporting activities (eg, jumping) so that the appendicular skeleton via the scapulothoracic junction and proximal hind limb musculature has a stable platform to attach to and optimally function.

Atrophy of the core stabilizing muscles has been documented due to pain and pathology and does not typically resolve until specific stabilizing exercises are implemented.[31] Measuring the cross-sectional area of the multifidus muscle allows for monitoring of disuse or neurogenic inhibition of the stabilizing muscles of the vertebral column. Stubbs and colleagues (2011)[32] developed dynamic mobilization exercises to target the multifidus muscle in horses (Video 1). The exercises were performed bilaterally for 5 repetitions, 5 days per week for 3 months, which produced a significant increase in multifidus cross-sectional area. The lateral bending component of the exercises toward the thoracolumbar and pelvic regions are most likely to target the multifidus and sacrocaudal muscles in the lumbosacral region.

The psoas minor muscle contributes to pelvic flexion with a fixed vertebral column and lumbosacral flexion when the pelvis is fixed. There have been no studies measuring activation of psoas minor possibly due to its deep location and relative inaccessibility. Considering the role of the psoas minor muscle, exercises that may activate the muscle are subtle caudal weight shifting, backing up a hill, pelvic flexion, and sternal elevation reflexes (see later discussion). The psoas minor muscle would also be recruited with dynamic mobilization exercises in lateral bending, as this exercise involves some lumbosacral flexion.

The ability to increase intraabdominal pressure is proposed as one of the key features of core stability.[28] The diaphragm serves a dual role as a muscle of respiration and to increase intraabdominal pressure.[33] The internal and external abdominal oblique and rectus abdominus muscles also support the abdominal viscera, increase intraabdominal pressure, and aid in expiration via the linked respiratory-locomotor cycle.[34] Trotting exercises[35] and walking and trotting over ground poles increase the activity of abdominal muscles.[36] The role of synchronized or coordinated movements of the diaphragm and the abdominal musculature in providing core stability is yet to be established in horses.

Specific Muscle Activation

The most reported clinical signs of sacroiliac joint pain and dysfunction is poor hind limb propulsion.[11] Therefore, targeting specific muscles that contribute to hind limb propulsion is often a focus of prescribed therapeutic exercises. The primary muscles involved in hind limb propulsion are as follows:

- Middle gluteal
- Biceps femoris
- Semimembranosus
- Semitendinosus

A common clinical finding is a lack of muscle development or atrophy of the vertebral portion of the biceps femoris muscle. To specifically activate this portion of the biceps femoris muscle, induced caudal weight shifting is applied at the diagonal forelimb during stance to induce contralateral pelvic stabilization. Contraction of the biceps femoris muscle can be observed or palpated to ensure optimal activation. An alternative method to activate specific muscles is to apply neuromuscular electrical stimulation (see later discussion).

Functional Muscle Activation

Functional muscle activation involves coordinated contraction of both the stabilizing and the global muscles of the pelvis, trunk, and limbs.[5] Functional muscle activation can be achieved with the following:

- Reflex responses to palpatory pressure
  - Pelvic flexion reflex (sustained or rhythmic) (Video 2)
  - Sternal elevation reflex (Video 3)
  - Sternal elevation reflex combined with lateral bending of the trunk (**Fig. 4**)
- Use of gymnastic equipment (Videos 4 and 5)[37]
  - Ground poles
  - Raised poles
  - Poles on a circle
  - Poles on slopes

The ground pole exercises may be performed at different gaits, usually at the walk and trot.

- Additional functional exercises
  - Lateral tail pulls—applied statically while standing or at a walking
  - Walking up and down inclines
  - Backing up a slope (Video 6)

Functional exercises have been combined with dynamic mobilization exercises applied 3 times per week for 6 weeks, which produced an increase in the cross-sectional area of the multifidus muscle.[38] The functional exercises included normal riding activities and gymnastic exercises, which included backing up, pelvic flexion reflexes, tight turns around a barrel, and walking over raised poles.

Training Aids

Training aids can be used to assist the functional movements of hind limb protraction and core stability.

- The Equiband system consists of an elasticized hindquarter and an abdominal band that stimulates activation of the abdominal and hind limb muscles and has a reported positive effect on dynamic stabilization of the trunk.[39] The Equiband system can be used in a functional and specific manner either in hand, on a lunge, or when a horse is ridden.[39]
- Theraband resistance bands can also be used in a similar way to Equiband to cause engagement of the hind limb and trunk musculature (**Fig. 5**).

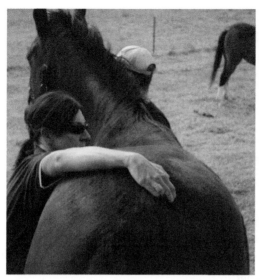

Fig. 4. Combined left lateral bending and flexion of the trunk. The practitioner's left hand is stimulating the girth region to induce elevation of the trunk, and the right hand is stimulating the contralateral sacral region to induce lateral bending.

Physical Modalities

Physical modalities can also be used to assist specific or functional muscle activities.

- Therapeutic elastic tape has been suggested to enhance proprioception via stimulation of superficial mechanoreceptors within the epidermis. There is a growing body of literature supporting the use of elastic tape in humans[40,41]; however, studies in normal horses have shown no clinical effects.[42]
- Further research is required to evaluate the effect of elastic tape on horses with movement deficits. Elastic tape may be used in combination with any form of therapeutic exercise with the intent of enhancing motor control for that specific task (**Fig. 6**).
- Neuromuscular electrical stimulation (NMES) may be used to stimulate dysfunctional or atrophied muscles. NMES is commonly used to activate and simulate voluntary muscle contractions.[43] NMES differs from voluntary muscle contraction, as it recruits motor units in a nonselective, spatially fixed, and temporally synchronous pattern (**Box 1**).[43]

Box 1
Neuromuscular electrical stimulation

NMES may be used
- In a static setting, where atrophied muscles are targeted in isolation (Video 7).
- In conjunction with therapeutic exercises. For example, caudal weight shifting to induce biceps femoris muscle activation as described earlier combined with electrodes placed over the affected muscle region with the applied electrical stimulation timed to induce muscle contraction at the same time as the applied caudal weight shifting.
- At slow gaits. For example, when walking over ground poles and other exercises such as backing up an incline.

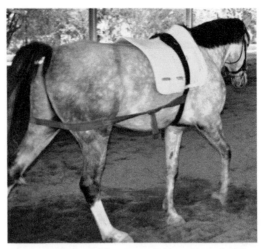

Fig. 5. Elastic therapeutic band attached to a surcingle and used to engage the hind limbs.

Interpreting Outcomes

When introducing a therapeutic exercise, training aid, or physical modality, the desired effect should be confirmed before progressing with further exercises or treatment. There are few validated outcome measures for evaluating the specific effects of therapeutic exercises in horses other than kinematic analysis of changes in stride length or vertebral displacement. Outcome measures used should be task related and functionally based.[9] Owners and trainers need to be educated to demonstrate effective

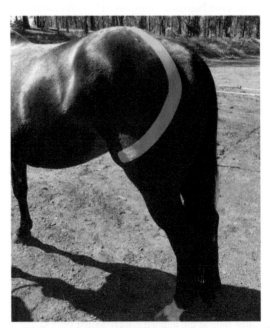

Fig. 6. Elastic therapeutic tape applied over the biceps femoris muscle from the origin to one of its insertions at the stifle. The tape was applied before performing therapeutic exercises in-hand.

delivery of the prescribed therapeutic exercise program and to also correctly interpret the desired outcome of the exercises.[9] Education and effective communication with owners and trainers is important in prescribing any therapeutic exercise.

If the desired clinical outcomes are not progressing as predicted, then the clinician should

1. Reevaluate the clinical reasoning process that originally identified the sacroiliac joint issues
2. Ensure that it is a functional instability requiring therapeutic exercise versus a more hypomobile, degenerative-type presentation
3. Reevaluate the specificity of the therapeutic exercise prescribed—is it specific to the task and the capability of the horse?

Rehabilitation of Sacroiliac Joint Hypomobility

Goals for managing sacroiliac joint hypomobility
- Attempt to restore lumbosacral and sacroiliac joint mobility
- Ensure adequate motion at the lumbosacral junction
- Attempt to restore global movements that could be secondarily limited (eg, hind limb protraction)
- Once the aforementioned goals are achieved then a therapeutic exercise program to improve motor control may be implemented

If the primary clinical signs indicate stiffness and a lack of mobility at the sacroiliac and lumbosacral joints (possibly due to more advanced degenerative processes), then the therapeutic approach is slightly modified to restore articular mobility and overall movement patterns. Restoring joint mobility via manual therapy techniques that incorporate baited stretches, active and passive mobilization, and manipulation may be sufficient to achieve functional movements. However, once normal sacroiliac joint movement is restored, the therapeutic exercise program should focus on improving motor control issues using the same principles as described earlier for functional instability. If severe degenerative changes in the sacroiliac joints exist,[20] then it may be difficult to restore optimal sacroiliac joint motion in affected horses, and as such they will always be a therapeutic challenge.

SUMMARY

Therapeutic exercise, combined with pain management, is one of the ways in which practitioners can manage altered patterns of muscle recruitment in horses with sacroiliac joint pain and dysfunction. When addressing muscle recruitment and motor control issues, activation and synchrony of the stabilizing muscles and the global or locomotor muscles need to be evaluated and treated based on the needs of the individual equine athlete. The prescription of therapeutic exercises must be specific and closely monitored to assess efficacy and desired outcome parameters within individual patients.

CLINICS CARE POINTS

- Clinician should establish if the sacroiliac dysfunction is related to hypermobility involving decreased motor control, or hypomobility involving degenerative change and fibrosis
- The clinician should ascertain if here is pain in the sacroiliac joint, related to the dysfunction
- Rehabilitation of sacroiliac joint dysfunction should be guided by the above

DISCLOSURE

The author has nothing to disclose.

SUPPLEMENTARY DATA

Supplementary data related to this article can be found online at https://doi.org/10.1016/j.cveq.2022.07.002.

REFERENCES

1. Chang L, Marsten G, Martin A. Anatomy, cartilage. Treasure Island (FL): Stat-Pearls [Internet] StatPearls Publishing; 2021.
2. Degueurce c, Chateau H, Denoix J. In vitro assessment of movements of the sacroiliac joint in the horse. Equine Vet J 2004;36:694–8.
3. Goff L, Jasiewicz J, Jeffcott L. Movement between the equine ilium and sacrum: in-vivo and in-vitro studies. Equine Vet J 2006;38(suppl):457–61.
4. Denoix J. Spinal biomechanics and functional anatomy. Vet Clin N Am Equine Pract 1999;15:27–50.
5. O'Sullivan P, Beales D, Beetham J, et al. Altered motor control strategies in subjects with sacroiliac joint pain during the active straight-leg raise-test. Spine 2002;27:E1–8.
6. Dyson S, Murray R. Pain associated with the sacroiliac joint region: a clinical study of 74 horses. Equine Vet J 2003;35:240–5.
7. Barstow A, Dyson S. Clinical features and diagnosis of sacroiliac joint region pain in 296 horses: 2004-2014. Equine Vet Educ 2015;27:637–47.
8. Laslett M. Evidence based diagnosis and treatment of the painful sacroiliac joint. J Man Manip Ther 2008;16:142–52.
9. McGowan C, Hyytiainen H. Muscular and neuromotor control and learning in the athletic horse. Comp Ex Phys 2017;13:185–94.
10. Vleeming A, Schuenke M, Masi A. The sacroiliac joint: an overview of its anatomy, function and potential clinical implications. J Anat 2012;221:537–67.
11. Jeffcott L, Dalin G, Ekman S, et al. Sacroiliac lesions as a cause of chronic poor performance in horses. Equine Vet J 1985;17:111–8.
12. Panjabi M. The stabilizing system of the spine. Part II. Neutral zone and stability hypothesis. J Spinal Disord 1992;5:390–6.
15. Felson D, Gale D, Elon Gale M, et al. Osteophytes and progression of knee osteoarthritis. Rheumatology 2005;44:100–4.
13. Panjabi M. A hypothesis of chronic back pain: ligament subfailure injuries lead to muscle control dysfunction. Eur Spine J 2006;668–76.
14. Yue J, Timm J, Panjabi M, et al. Clinical application of the Panjabi neutral zone hypothesis: the Stabilomax NZ posterior dynamic lumbar stabilization system. Neurosurg Focus 2007;22:E12. https://doi.org/10.3171/foc.2007.22.1.12.
16. Sangwan S, Green R, Taylor N. Characteristics of stabilizer muscles: a systematic review. Physiother Can 2014;66:348–58.
17. Arokoski J, Valta T, Airaksinen O, et al. Back and abdominal muscle function during stabilization exercises. Arch Phys Med Rehabil 2001;82:1089–98.
18. Krishnan Y, Grodzinsky A. Cartilage diseases. Matrix Biol 2018;71-72:51–69.
19. Takahashi I, Matsuzaki T, Yoshida S, et al. Difference in cartilage repair between loading and unloading environments in the rat knee. J Jpn Phys Ther Assoc 2014;17:22–30.
20. Goff L, Jeffcott L, Riggs C, et al. Sacroiliac joint morphology: influence of age, body weight and previous back pain. Equine Vet J 2014;46:52.

21. Haussler K, Stover S, Willits N. Pathological change in lumbosacral vertebrae and pelvis in thoroughbred racehorses. Am J Vet Res 1999;60:143–53.
22. Monticone M, Barbarino A, Testi C, et al. Symptomatic efficacy of stabilizing treatment versus laser therapy for sub-acute low back pain with positive tests for sacroiliac dysfunction: a randomised clinical controlled trial with 1 year follow-up. Euro Medicophys 2004;40:263–8.
23. Visser I, Woudenberg N, de Bont J, et al. Treatment of the sacroiliac joint in patients with leg pain: a randomized controlled trial. Eur Spine J 2013;22:2310–7.
24. Heinricher M, Tavares I, Leith J, et al. Descending control of nociception: specificity, recruitment and plasticity. Brain Res Rev 2009;60:214–25.
25. Burkholder T, Lieber R. Sarcomere length operating range of vertebrate muscles during movement. J Exp Biol 2001;204:1529–36.
26. Gronwald T, Torpel A, Herold F, et al. Perspective of dose and response for individualised physical exercise and training prescription. J Funct Morphol Kinesiol 2020;5. https://doi.org/10.3390/jfmk5030048.
27. Ameli S, Naghdy F, Stirling D, et al. Quantitative and non-invasive measurement of exercise induced fatigue. J Sports Eng Technology 2019;233:34–45.
28. Akuthota V, Nalder S. Core Strengthening. Arch Phys Med Rehabil 2004;85:586–92.
29. Bliven K, Anderson B. Core stability training for injury prevention. Sports Health 2013;514–22.
30. Stubbs N, Hodges P, Jeffcott L, et al. Functional anatomy of the caudal thoracolumbar and lumbosacral spine in the horse. Equine Vet J Suppl 2006;36:393–9.
31. Hides J, Richardson C, Jull G. Multifidus muscle recovery is not automatic following resolution of acute first episode low level pain. Spine 1996;21:2763–9.
32. Stubbs N, Kaiser L, Hauptman J, et al. Dynamic mobilisation exercises increase cross-sectional area of musculus multifidus. Equine Vet J 2011;43:522–9.
33. Fogarty M, Sieck G. Evolution and functional differentiation of the diaphragm muscles of mammals. Compr Physiol 2020;9:715–66.
34. Jones K. New insights on equid locomotor evolution from the lumbar region of fossil horses. Proc R Soc B 2016;283:20152947.
35. Zsoldos R, Kotschwar A, Kotschwar AB. Activity of the equine rectus abdominis and oblique external abdominal muscles measured by surface EMG at the walk and trot on the treadmill. Equine Vet J 2010;42:S523–9.
36. Shaw K, Ursini T, Levine D. Longissimus dorsi and rectus abdominus muscle activity during equine walk and trot. JEVS 2021;107.
37. Murray R, Walker V, MacKechnie-Guire R, et al. Effect of walking over ground poles and raised poles compared to no poles on limb and back kinematics in horses with different postures. Equine Vet J 2020;52:1–17.
38. de Oliveira K, Soutello R, da Fonsesca R, et al. Gymnastic training and dynamic mobilisation exercises improved stride quality and increase epaxial muscle size in therapy horses. JEVS 2015;35:888–93.
39. Pfau T, Simons F, Rombach N, et al. Effect of 4-week elastic resistance band training regimen on back kinematics in horses trotting in-hand and on the lunge. Equine Vet J 2017;49:823–35.
40. Kelle B, Guzel R, Sakalli H. The effect of kinesio-taping application for acute non-specific low back pain: a randomized controlled clinical trial. Clin Rehab 2016;30:997–1003.

41. Ericson C, Stenfeldt P, Hardeman A. Effect of kinesiotape on flexion-extension of the thoracolumbar back in horses at trot. Animals 2020;10:301.
42. Cho H, Kim E, Kim Y, et al. Kinesio taping improves pain, range of motion, and proprioception in older patients with knee osteoarthritis. Am J Phys Med Rehabil 2015;94:192–200.
43. Bickel S, Gregory C, Dean J. Motor unit recruitment during neuromuscular electrical stimulation - a critical appraisal. Eur J App Phys 2011;111: 2399–4072011.

Tack Fit and Use

Hilary M. Clayton, BVMS, PhD[a,b,]*, Russell MacKechnie-Guire, PhD[c,d]

KEYWORDS

- Saddle • Bridle • Bit • Equestrian sport • Pressure • Pain • Atrophy

KEY POINTS

- A variety of equipment is used by riders to facilitate control of the horse.
- Equipment should fit correctly and be effective but not coercive.
- Signs of ill-fit or misuse of equipment should be recognized.
- Familiarity with correction of tack fitting problems is beneficial.

INTRODUCTION

Tack is used to improve safety, comfort, and communication between the rider and horse. In order to accomplish this, the bit, bridle, saddle, and girth should be fitted and used correctly. Ill-fitting tack and insensitive and asymmetric application of the rider's aids transmitted via the tack may cause a variety of lesions, such as ulceration and bruising, that interfere with equine health and athletic performance. The saddle needs to fit the size, shape, and contours of the horse's back on its underside and the rider's pelvis and thighs on the upper side. The change in back contours from the relatively upright slope visualized along the lateral aspect of the withers to the more horizontal orientation beneath the rider's seat is accommodated by the twist of the saddle, which is one of several contributing factors to consider for correct saddle fit and the horse's comfort. The bridle is designed primarily to hold the bit in place and should not be used to apply extraneous pressure over sensitive tissues of the head by incorrect placement, lack of padding, or overtightening of the bridle straps (nosebands/headpieces). The size, type, and height of the bit relative to the oral cavity dimensions determines its contact with the horse's lips and commissures, bars, tongue, and hard palate. Oral lesions caused by bits may vary from commissural ulcers associated with snaffle bits or lesions of the bars related to unjointed bits (snaffle or curb). The rider can affect the development of skin lesions or injuries via their weight

[a] Department of Large Animal Clinical Sciences, College of Veterinary Medicine, Michigan State University, 736 Wilson Road, East Lansing, MI 48824, USA; [b] Sport Horse Science, LLC, 3145 Sandhill Road, Mason, MI 48854, USA; [c] Hartpury University, Hartpury House, Gloucester, Gloucestershire, GL 19 3BE, United Lingdom; [d] Centaur Biomechanics, LTD, Dunstaffanage House, Moreton Morrell, Warwickshire, CV35 9BD, United Kingdom
* Corresponding author. 3145 Sandhill Road, Mason, MI 48854.
E-mail address: claytonh@msu.edu

Vet Clin Equine 38 (2022) 585–601
https://doi.org/10.1016/j.cveq.2022.07.003
0749-0739/22/© 2022 Elsevier Inc. All rights reserved.

distribution in the saddle, ability to ride in harmony with the horse, and skill in applying light and consistent aids.

Challenges inherent in correct fitting and use of equipment are similar across disciplines and center around the following principles:

- Saddle fit should allow unhindered back and shoulder movement
- The saddle needs to accommodate changes in the shape of the horse's back over time
- The bridle should fit and be adjusted correctly, particularly with regard to noseband tightness
- Oral lesions are often present in sport horses and warrant greater awareness and understanding
- Coercive riding techniques should not be condoned

THE SADDLE

Saddles were developed primarily to improve comfort of the horse by distributing the rider's weight over the horse's back. Safety was also an important factor by providing the rider with a more stable platform on which to ride the horse. Saddle design should address the following:

- Account for the disparate shapes of the horse's back versus the rider's pelvis and inner thighs
- Allow for shape changes of the horse (and perhaps the rider) over time
- Correct fit in the static and dynamic horse
- The bones and muscles of the horse's shoulders and back need to move beneath the saddle
- The saddle's balance on the horse's back
- The rider's ability to ride in harmony with the horse

From the horse's standpoint, the saddle should support three-dimensional movements of the subcutaneous musculoskeletal tissues and scapula, including the superficial scapular and trunk muscles, and the thoracic vertebrae and ribs.

The following text describes the structure and fitting of an English saddle. Most English saddles are built around a tree that provides a degree of rigidity and a mechanism to distribute the forces due to the rider. Modern trees have a little flexibility to accommodate movements of the horse's back. The pommel and cantle refer to the elevated areas at the front and back, respectively, of the saddle. The panels on the underside form the interface between the saddle and the horse's back and are padded to accommodate the changing contours of the back and help to distribute and reduce saddle pressures.

Different groups have slightly different recommendations for saddle fitting. The Society of Master Saddlers, a certificated society in saddle and bridle fit, provides the following guidelines for fitting a saddle to a static horse:

1. General feel of the saddle
2. Width and shape of the head plate closely matches the contours of the horse
3. Correct tree positioning with the scapula free to rotate
4. Weight-bearing part of the panel does not extend beyond T18
5. The gullet clears the spinous process of the withers and midline of the back
6. Girth straps align with the girth groove
7. Saddle is balanced craniocaudally and stable laterally
8. Panels have smooth, consistent contact with the horse's back

9. Rider fit

Assessment is subjective and for some criteria, trained saddle fitters do not show a good level of agreement in assessing the adequacy of saddle fit.[1] Notably, features that are not visible externally, particularly those related to the angle of the tree points (tree width) and tree length are the most difficult to assess. It was also found that saddler height was a limiting factor with saddlers who were short in stature having more difficulty in accurately assessing saddle fit.

Observation of the horse's back from above shows how back shape changes within the saddle contact region. On either side of the withers, the trunk slopes quite steeply downward over the lateral chest wall but in the mid-to-caudal thoracic region, the slope is more horizontal. This change in contour is accommodated by the twist in the saddle tree where the underside changes from a relatively narrow V-shape over the withers to a broader, flatter shape behind the withers. This changing contour is one of the more difficult aspects to evaluate while assessing proper saddle fit. A saddle with a narrow twist can create localized bilateral pressures in the epaxial muscles at the level of T10-T13. These pressures were of sufficient magnitude to affect gait when trotting,[2] jumping,[3] and galloping.[4] When pressures were reduced with saddlery modifications, gait features were altered, highlighting the importance of correct saddle fit and the effect that areas of high pressures induced by saddle design can have on equine locomotion.

The head plate of the English saddle is the rigid element that connects the left and right sides of the tree and forms the elevated front portion of the saddle (ie, pommel; **Fig. 1**). Its width and angulation should correspond to the shape of the dorsal wither region with proper width at the apex to provide clearance of the spinous processes and outward angulation of the points to provide uniform contact and weight distribution of the rider. Wither conformation may change with age and level of training, so fit of the head plate and saddle must be checked periodically.

If the head plate is too wide or the angle is too large (**Fig. 2**), the saddle will not be sufficiently supported and the tree will slide down and place abnormal pressure on the top of the withers, with a tendency for pressure to be concentrated along the caudal border of the scapula[5] and create localized bilateral pressures in the epaxial muscle lateral to T10-T13. When the saddle is removed, the presence of dry patches of

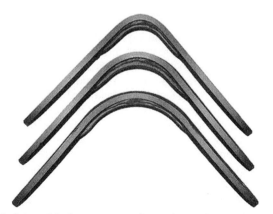

Fig. 1. Three head plates with the same overall angulation but with different apex widths and shapes. The lower part of the tree points, which are within the panels, should match the curvature of the horse's back. (Courtesy WOW Saddles.)

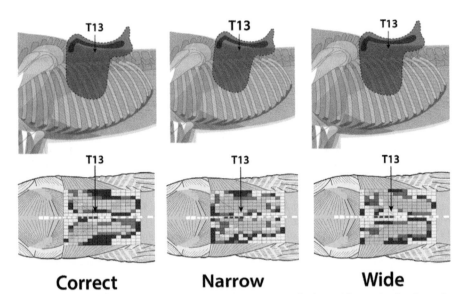

Correct   Narrow   Wide

Fig. 2. Saddle positions (*above*) and typical pressure scans (*below* with 4 red cells along the midline of the pad) for, left to right, a saddle correctly fitted (*left*), too narrow (*middle*), and too wide (*right*). The correctly fitted saddle on the left shows a fairly even pressure pattern on the horse's back. The narrow saddle (*center*) has the pommel high, the cantle low, and the seat slopes backward. The narrow saddle can bridge, causing 4 high-pressure areas (*red and yellow colors* in the pressure scans): 2 cranially and 2 caudally. The wide saddle (*right*) is low in the pommel high in the cantle, and the seat tilts forward and downward. Localized high-pressure areas are seen cranially on each side of the withers in the accompanying pressure scan. Cranial to the left in all images.

skin on the side(s) of the withers surrounded by normal sweat patterns reflects saddle pressure sufficient to cause sweat gland ischemia.[6] Localized muscle pain and concavities in the epaxial muscles (trapezius, rhomboideus thoracis, longissimus dorsi) may be palpable in the affected area soon after exercise and over time. An excessively wide head plate may drop low enough to apply direct pressure to the spinous processes of the withers.

If the head plate is too narrow or its angle is too small, the pommel of the saddle will be visibly elevated with the saddle appearing to be tilted backward. A common observation with a narrow tree is bridging in which there are 4 points of pressure. Bilateral areas of localized high pressures in the epaxial muscles, lateral to T10-T13 and caudal to the scapula (longissimus, cutaneus trunci, latissimus, deep pectoral) can often be found due to the narrow saddle. Due to the "bridging" bilateral pressures are also concentrated in the region lateral to T16-T18. The cranial-caudal pressure pattern induced by a narrow saddle can span from the medial part of the long back muscles[5] and laterally. The mid-thoracic part of the back is a relatively unloaded area between (see **Fig. 2**). Physical examination may show signs of muscle pain or atrophy in the heavily loaded areas. Both wide and narrow saddles may negatively affect trunk function and limb movement patterns.[7]

The twist of the tree should match the horse's back contours to accommodate the three-dimensional change in angle between the withers and the back. A horse with a narrow back needs a saddle with a narrow twist and vice versa. The rider's preference for more or less support between their upper thighs should be regarded as a secondary concern. Correctly fitted saddles that have a narrow twist have been associated with high pressures at T10-T13 (**Fig. 3**) that affect limb movement when trotting,[2] jumping,[3] and galloping.[4] Horses develop locomotor strategies to alter the area of weight-bearing on the back with the goal of alleviating discomfort caused by saddle-induced pressures.[2] Fortunately, these altered gait parameters can be improved with proper saddle fit modifications to reduce pressure at T10-T13.

The panels of the saddle provide the main surface contact area with the horse and should match the contours of the horse's back both cranial-to-caudal and left-to-right when viewed from behind (**Fig. 4**). If the horse has epaxial muscle atrophy or a generalized lack of muscle development and the panels are too flat, there can be a localized band of high pressure located close to the dorsal midline. If the panels slope more than the horse's back, pressure increases along the periphery of the panels.[5]

Panels vary in size, shape, flocking material used, and in their firmness, which affects the interface with and comfort of the horse. The traditional flocking material is wool, which optimally should be reflocked every few months as the horse's back shape changes and the flocking can be compressed and become hard and lumpy within the panels. Foam panels may retain their shape for a long period of time and depending on the type of foam used (closed cell) they do not disintegrate over time. However, foam is more difficult to adjust than wool. Air-flocked panels with a foam core are another option so long as they are not overinflated, which makes the panels hard and causes the back of the saddle to bounce in gaits with suspension phases pitching the cranial part of the saddle downward to create localized, high pressure areas. When inflated properly, air panels are soft and conform easily to the changing shape of the underlying bones and muscles.

The underside of the panels should be smooth without focal hard or raised areas and the edges of the panels should curve gently. The gullet should be of uniform width along the length of the saddle (see **Fig. 4**). In horses with an elongated wither conformation, the upper part of the gullet of the saddle may contact the spinous processes on the caudal slope of the withers. If the hair over the top or caudal slope of the withers seems ruffled when the saddle is removed, the gullet width and clearance should be checked along the entire length of the saddle. Consideration should also be given to the saddle pad being used as this may displace ventrally during locomotion.

Modular saddles with interchangeable parts are available and can be assembled stall-side so that the size and shape of the tree, the length, width, and depth of the

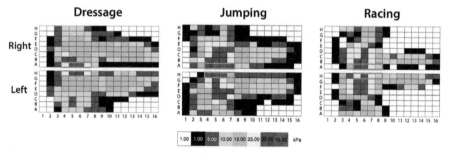

Fig. 3. High-pressure areas at the twist of the saddle are shown by pink, red, and yellow shaded cells on the pressure scan in a dressage saddle (*left*), a jumping saddle (*center*) and a full tree racing saddle (*right*). The twist of the saddle corresponds to the narrowest part of the saddle at the region of T10-13. If the twist is too narrow for the horse, it can cause localized pressures in this region, which can affect gait. Cranial to the left.

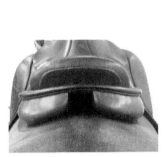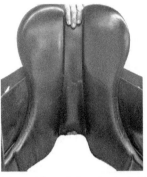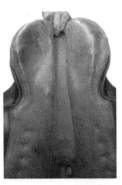

Fig. 4. Left: Rear view of a saddle with a wide gullet and panels that curve gently away from the side of the horse. Center: Underside of a foam-flocked saddle showing smooth, wide panels and wide gullet. Right: Underside of a saddle with lumpy panels and inconsistent gullet width.

panels, and the size and shape of the seat can be customized to fit the horse and rider as needed over time. This is particularly useful when fitting a young horse or one that is rehabilitating and can be expected to dramatically change the shape of the dorsal trunk.

When the horse is in motion, the saddle may move slightly craniocaudally in rhythm with the footfalls. The rider's seat and the saddle should, on average, be positioned centrally on the horse's back, although there may be some lateral motion of the back of the saddle coinciding with specific moments in each gait. The rider's seat and the caudal portion of the saddle have been reported to show consistent asymmetric or excessive displacement to one side, which is sometimes referred to as "saddle slip." Asymmetric lateral displacement of the caudal portion of the saddle has been related to hindlimb lameness, with the saddle being displaced more toward the lame or lamer hindlimb. Symmetric saddle kinematics were restored when the source of lameness was alleviated.[8] Another study reported asymmetric saddle displacement in 24% of horses with hindlimb lameness alone, 46% of horses with concurrent fore and hind limb lameness, and 5% with forelimb lameness suggesting a relationship to hind limb lameness, with or without concurrent forelimb lameness with the overarching finding that asymmetric movement of the horse (here: lameness) may affect the balance of the saddle causing it to slip to one side. Not all lame horses have saddle slip and not all nonlame horses have a saddle that remains straight. Other factors associated with saddle slip include functional/structural asymmetry of the horse that is not associated with lameness. In these horses, the primary factor(s) responsible for the saddle slipping to the side are unknown. The consensus seems to be that the horse, not the rider, is the primary causative factor; asymmetrical riders were found not to induce saddle slip.[8,9]

When the caudal portion of the saddle is displaced to one side (eg, to the right), saddle pressure increases on the contralateral (left) side in the soft tissues lateral to the midline in the region of T10-T13 and more caudally at T17-T18 (**Fig. 5**). Saddle slip only happens on one rein and generally more noticeably in walk and canter largely due to the inherent rotations of the horse's back in these gaits. It may be accompanied by asymmetries of limb movement due to changes in the rider's center of pressure and balance, together with asymmetric saddle pressures. During ridden locomotion, when the saddle slips to one side, the rider's pelvis follows the saddle while the rider's trunk

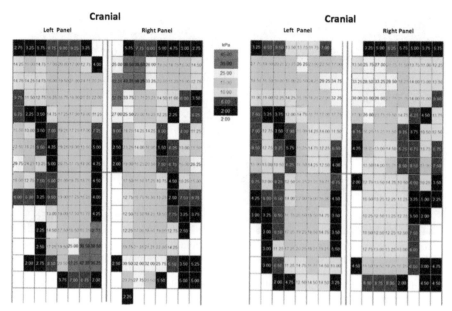

Fig. 5. Left: Pressure scan of a saddle with excessive displacement of the caudal portion of the saddle to the left with corresponding increased pressure close to the midline at the front of the saddle on the right side when in left lead canter; Right: Pressure map of the same horse and rider after saddle slip was reduced by the insertion of a shim and changing the girthing arrangement to rebalance the saddle.

compensates by leaning away from the direction of saddle displacement. In general, saddle pressure is higher on the side that the rider's leans toward.[10] As a way of determining if the horse is the primary cause of saddle slip, when walking in a straight-line without a rider, the saddle will persistently slip to one side. When the rider mounts, the saddle will follow the same movement as when walking in a straight-line without the rider.

As a temporary mechanical intervention, a saddle fitter may use asymmetric shims or flocking to alleviate areas of high pressures caused by saddle slip or use a different billet strap attachment or arrangement to temporarily correct or reduce slippage while the underlying cause is remedied. After eliminating lameness, an exercise program should be used to strengthen the horse and reduce the effect of existing functional and structural asymmetries. Riders also need to consider their own position and asymmetries; prolonged riding in a saddle that displaces to one side may have affected their functional riding ability.

Sometimes, it is difficult to find a saddle that fits both horse and rider. Some riders may choose to use treeless saddles that are purported to offer a more universal fit but, without a tree, pressure tends to be concentrated in small areas on the horse's back[11] **(Fig. 6)**. Horses ridden in treeless saddles may have focal painful areas in the epaxial musculature at T13-T17, which corresponds to the riders contact points (seat bones). Additional padding beneath the saddle may be helpful to reduce peak pressures but the duration or intensity of ridden exercise, the rider's ability, and the athletic discipline may also be factors to consider. Some treeless saddles have the stirrup leathers suspended by a continuous band across the horse's back, which may cause localized pressures and back soreness directly over the dorsal midline.

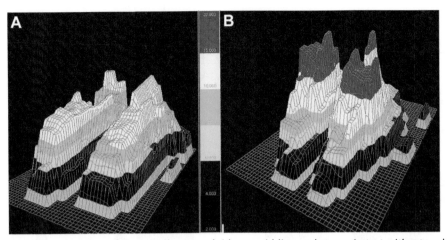

Fig. 6. Pressure maps of the same horse and rider at middiagonal stance in trot with a treed saddle (A) and a treeless saddle (B). The area of the pressure mat is shown by the white squares with the colors and heights of the individual rectangular cells on the pressure scan indicating pressure magnitude. Note the higher peak forces distributed over a smaller area for the treeless saddle.

BRIDLES

The basic English bridle consists of a headpiece and cheekpieces to support the bit, a browband, noseband, throatlatch or jowl strap, bit and reins. Similar to proper saddle fitting, the principles of pressure reduction in bridles include increasing the weight-bearing areas and adding soft padding to the underside. Firm padding is much less effective in dampening force. The padding should be easily indented by digital pressure. One bridle features a thick layer of padding that consists of material used to reduce the risk of bedsores in humans, which compresses and self-adjusts to the horse's head when tightened in place. A current trend is to use "anatomic" bridles intended to relieve pressure over sensitive areas of the head and poll region. The common features of an anatomic bridle are illustrated in **Fig. 7.** Other bridles apply similar principles but with variations in design and esthetics.

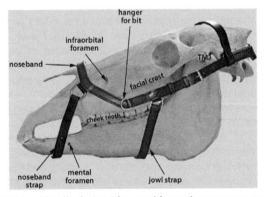

Fig. 7. Anatomic (Micklem) bridle designed to avoid exerting pressure on sensitive anatomic structures labeled on the diagram. TMJ, temporomandibular joint.

The ears and adjacent poll region are sensitive. Pressure on the aural cartilages, the caudal auricular muscles, or neurovascular structures may cause signs of head tossing or shaking, an unsteady head carriage, unsteady contact with the bit, holding the head behind or ahead of the vertical, twisting at the poll, avoiding a consistent contact with the bit as well as more generalized signs of discomfort or resistance.[12] Note, however, that these signs of pain are not pathognomonic for poor bridle fit or use.

Things to consider around the ears:

- Many bridles have a cut out area for the ears, which is beneficial as long as the cut out is in the correct place for the individual horse (**Fig. 8**).
- If the browband is too short, it pulls the headpiece forward against the back of the ears; a too long browband is preferable over a too short browband.
- Some headpieces are designed to avoid pressure over the dorsal midline of the poll; however, pressure relief in one location inevitably increases pressure elsewhere. In this case, pressure increases on either side of the poll in the area behind the ears, which some horses find particularly painful.
- Research using a small pressure mat[13] indicated high pressure where the browband joins the headpiece. Cushioned pads on the headpiece provided clearance at the base of and ventral to the ear (**Fig. 9**).

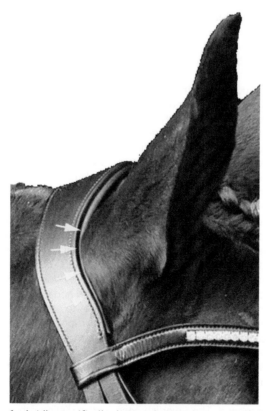

Fig. 8. Headpiece of a bridle specifically designed to contour around the caudal aspect of the external ear (*yellow arrows*) to relieve pressure applied on the back of the ears.

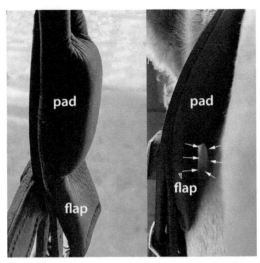

Fig. 9. Left: Caudal view of a cheekpiece of a bridle with an added foam pad and attached flap; right: the added padding lifts the cheekpiece away from the horse's face to relieve pressure in the area outlined by white arrows.

When using a leverage bit, conventional wisdom is that rein tension rotates the lower shank backward while the upper shank rotates forward and applies pressure via the cheekpiece and headpiece to the poll. However, the amount of poll pressure is actually considerably less than expected due to the elasticity of the horse's lips allowing the fulcrum to move.[14]

The cheekpiece should lie ventral to the facial crest, which means that the front part of the noseband must be long enough to allow for proper cheekpiece placement, which can be difficult in breeds with a prominent nasal region. Areas in which the bones of the skull are located superficially are vulnerable to bridle pressure. The buckles on the bridle should overly soft tissues, such as the masseter muscle rather than bones, particularly around the temporomandibular joint.

The throatlatch is intended to prevent the bridle falling off over the ears but it should not be tight enough to put excessive pressure on the ventral throat area when the poll is flexed. Some bridles use a jowl strap in addition to, or instead of, a throatlatch, which is more effective both in keeping the bridle on the horse's head and in preventing the cheekpiece from moving dorsally toward the facial crest (see **Fig. 7**).

The noseband is undoubtedly the most controversial part of the bridle. It is suspended from a strap that passes over the top of the head, or sometimes incorporated as part of the headpiece. One or 2 straps encircle the nose and mouth. A correctly adjusted noseband is used as an aid to help teach the horse to accept the bit without opening the mouth excessively, by allowing the jaws to separate by a small amount before the noseband tightens and applies supportive pressure to the muzzle region. When the mouth closes, a properly tensioned noseband should immediately release pressure, so it acts by negative reinforcement.

Some nosebands have a single strap and others, such as the flash and **Fig. 8** nosebands, have 2 straps going around the horse's face. When the noseband has a single strap fitted 1 to 2 cm below the facial crest, it may be classified as a cavesson or a Swedish (crank) noseband. The Swedish noseband is distinguished by having a double strap arrangement under the jaw that incorporates a padded chin piece to cushion the edges of the mandibles. It also usually has a well-padded area over the dorsum of the nose. A drop noseband has a single strap but is fitted lower on the face, just above the maxillary notch, and its ventral strap is fitted below the mouthpiece of the bit.

Lesions at the lip commissures have been related to tightness of the upper noseband strap, which is the one placed higher on the horse's head, and having a looser upper strap is significantly associated with fewer commissural lesions.[15] Without a noseband, however, the prevalence of lesions at the lip commissures increased 2.6 times compared with the loosest noseband category.[15] Neither the presence nor tightness of a lower noseband (flash, see **Fig. 8**, Micklem) affected the prevalence of lesions at the lip commissures[15] probably because the lower strap crosses the interdental space where teeth are absent.

When the noseband is overtightened, the areas sustaining the highest pressures are the lateral edges of the nasal bones and the underside of the mandible,[16] that is, the areas where the noseband runs over bony prominences.[13,16,17] An ingenious solution is a noseband with a foam pad over the bridge of the horse's nose that completely off loads the edges of the nasal bones[13] (**Fig. 10**).

Some riders overtighten the noseband to keep the horse's mouth closed, especially in sports that penalize the horse for opening its mouth or exteriorizing their tongue. Horses that habitually open their mouths when ridden are likely to be suffering intraoral pain or discomfort. These horses should be examined while wearing the bridle and noseband adjusted in the typical manner to evaluate whether the bridle fits and is adjusted correctly. The horse and rider may also be observed during ridden work to evaluate the rider's position and use of the reins and the horse's response, including resistant behaviors. After removing the bit and bridle, a perioral and intraoral examination should be performed to examine the lips, oral commissures, buccal mucosa, the bars, the tongue, and the hard palate for the presence of lesions or painful tissues. The dental arcades should be examined for overgrowths on the rostral cheek teeth and for the presence of wolf teeth and whether they are erupted or not. If a potentially painful oral lesion is found, the underlying cause should, if possible, be identified, and the lesion should be treated and allowed to heal before resuming exercise with the offending bit or bridle.

BITS

Perhaps, more than any other item of tack, new bits appear frequently on the market that incorporate reported changes in design or materials. The effects of the bit within

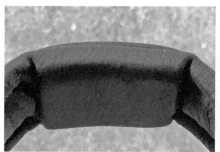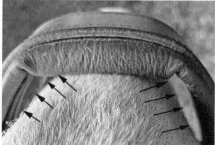

Fig. 10. Left: Inner surface of noseband showing a soft foam pad applied on the dorsal midline; right: the pad completely off-loads the left and right edges of the nasal bones (*black arrows*).

the oral cavity are difficult to evaluate visually but radiographic and fluoroscopic studies have provided information describing bit orientation and contact with intraoral structures.[18–21] When rein tension is applied, the orientation of the bit within the mouth does not change[22] but it may move relative to oral structures leading to increased or decreased pressure.

A bit consists of a mouthpiece that may be unjointed or include one or more joints. The mouthpiece attaches via rings on its lateral sides to the cheekpieces of the bridle and to the reins. A snaffle bit is a nonleverage bit with the cheekpiece and the rein attaching to the same ring. An exception to this is the hanging cheek (Baucher) snaffle in which the cheekpiece attaches above the rein, perhaps allowing a small amount of leverage. In a curb bit, the rein attaches to a shank (cheek) below the level of the mouthpiece and the cheekpiece attaches to a shorter shank above the mouthpiece. Rein tension may have a leverage effect by rotating the upper shank forward, increasing tension in the cheekpiece, and applying pressure to the poll.

The bit is interposed between the tongue and hard palate and, because the oral cavity is a virtual space,[18] the bit is accommodated within the malleable, muscular tissue of the tongue that molds around it.[18] When the horse's lips are parted, the tongue bulges out between the bars at the interdental space and acts as a cushion to protect the bars from bit pressure. The tongue can also push against the mouthpiece of the bit to relieve pressure.

The cheekpieces are adjusted so that the bit fits into the corners of the lips usually with a single fold or wrinkle of the lips. The commissures of the lips are the most common site of bit-related injuries, which include bruises or ulcers (**Fig. 11**) at the commissures and on the buccal mucosa. Horses ridden with a snaffle bit have 8 times higher risk for developing buccal lesions.[23]

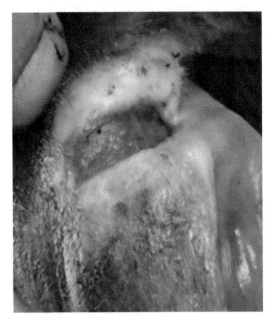

Fig. 11. Typical ulcer located in the lip commissure due to excessive bit pressure. (Photo courtesy of Dr. Mette Uldahl.)

Uldahl and colleagues[24] described in detail a protocol for analyzing and categorizing lesions of the oral commissures, including potentially pathologic changes in pigmentation, roughness, erosions, contusion, and scars. Applying this classification to horses at a precompetition evaluation[25], about 8% of horses examined had commissural ulcers indicating current damage and about 30% had scars indicating previous damage. Most types of lesions were bilateral (ulcers, scars, fissures, bruises). Although very few horses had isolated lesions on the bars, those horses with commissural erosions, bruises, and ulcers had similar lesions on the bars. Dental overgrowths (hooks, sharp enamel points) were usually bilateral but not related to mucosal ulcers or erosion or contusion at the lip commissures. However, ulcers around the lip commissures were associated with scarring and depigmentation in that area, which are evidence of previous bit damage. There was a clear relationship between the presence of current and previous perioral and intraoral damage indicating the ongoing nature of poor bit fit or use problems.

Studies in several sports have reported oral lesions in horses immediately after competition:

- In 3143 dressage horses, show jumpers, eventers, and endurance horses, 9% had oral lesions or blood at the lip commissures.[15]
  - Lesions increased with level of competition but did not differ between bit types or bitless bridles
  - A looser upper noseband had reduced risk of oral lesions but the absence of a cavesson increased the risk of commissural lesions 2 times compared with the loosest noseband
- Fifty-two percent of eventers had acute oral lesions immediately after cross-country.[26]
- Eighty-four percent of trotters had acute oral lesions after racing.[27]
  - Two percent were bleeding
  - Five percent had blood on the bit but not visible externally
- Racehorses wearing snaffle bits had a high prevalence of severe injuries of the lip commissures and bone spurs on the bars.[28]
- Polo ponies wearing gag bits had bone spurs on the bars and some had tongue ulcerations.[28]

Some horses play with the bit excessively using their tongue to raise the mouthpiece and grasp it between the premolars,[19] especially when using jointed bits. Unjointed mouthpieces lie higher on the tongue (**Fig. 12**) and have less intraoral mobility than jointed bits, which hang with the joint(s) lower on the tongue, especially if the mouthpiece is too wide or the cheekpieces are too long.[19] In these cases, check the following:

- The width of the bit should be about 1 cm wider than the distance between the lip commissures.
- The bit should be adjusted to fit into the commissures of the lips with a small wrinkle present in the skin.

In double-jointed bits, the width of the central link determines the position of the joints relative to the bars (**Fig. 13**). If the central link is narrow, the joints are less likely to be directly over the bars. If the joints are directly over the bars, there is the potential for the loops of the joint to press against the bars. Some bit designs are intended to be inserted into the horse's mouth in a specific orientation to ensure the loops lie parallel to the bars. If these bits are negligently or deliberately reversed, the loops of the joint will be perpendicular to the bars, which increase the potential for pain and injury.

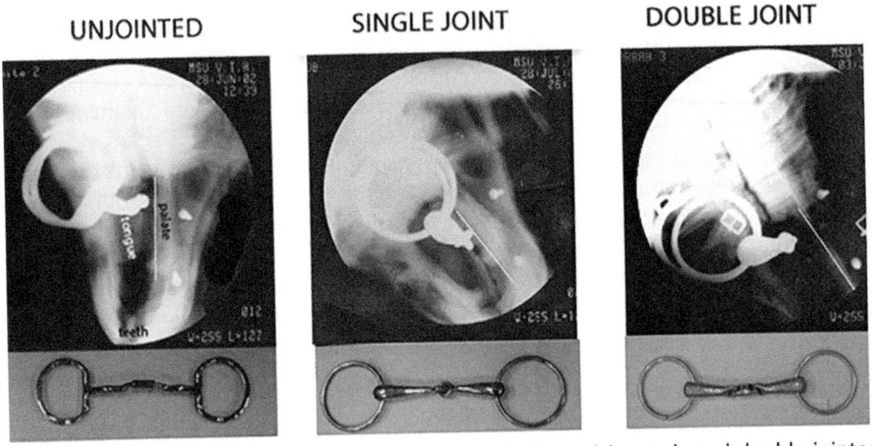

UNJOINTED   SINGLE JOINT   DOUBLE JOINT

Fig. 12. Lateral radiographs of unjointed (*left*), single-jointed (*center*), and double-jointed (*right*) snaffle bits. Dorsal to the right. Yellow line shows position of the hard palate. Note how far the bits hang down on the tongue in each image, which can be assessed by the distance from the most rostral part of the bit to the rostral edge of the first cheek tooth. Note also the proximity of the 3 bits to the line representing the hard palate.

For many years, it was thought that thicker mouthpieces were kinder because they distributed pressure over a larger area but it is now recognized that bits of medium diameter (14–17 mm measured at the outer edge) are associated with fewer lesions.[26] Large diameter bits are too big to fit into the limited space between the bars, whereas thin bits are more likely to localize pressure and cause damage.

The bit type affects the lesion type. Bruises, ulcers, and bone spurs on the bars are usually associated with unjointed (curb) bits, with horses ridden in ported curb bits

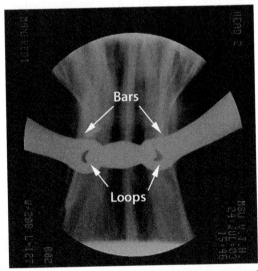

Fig. 13. Dorsoventral radiograph showing the relationship between the mouthpiece of a double-jointed bit and the bars of the mandible. Note the canons of the mouthpiece extending laterally on either side of the bars. The bars are separated from the lip commissures by a distance of several centimetres[31] due to the intervening fleshy cheeks and narrowing of the mandible in this area.

being 75 times more likely to have lesions on the bars.[23] It has been suggested that curb bits with a large, backward-sloping tongue relief or port are most likely to cause these lesions. When rein tension rotates the lower shank backward, the port rotates forward against the palate and the mouthpiece presses down on the bars. If the port is angled forward relative to the shanks, it does not impinge on the hard palate. A large tongue relief or port allows the tongue to bulge into the elevation but makes it more difficult for the horse to push against the bit to reduce pressure. Bit-related damage to the tongue is infrequent and is usually associated with severe damage to the bars caused by an unjointed bit.

The hard palate seems particularly sensitive to pressure. There are intraindividual differences between horses in the shape (flat or arched), width (34–50 mm), and height (5–14 mm) of the palate,[29] and these are likely to influence the risk of bit contact. Palate contact is usually from the loops of a jointed snaffle or from a port that is oriented backward (caudally) relative to the shanks. When rein tension rotates the port into the palatine tissues, horses respond by opening the mouth to reduce palate pressure.[19] Riders may respond by overtightening the noseband.

Bit-associated lesions bleed infrequently, although blood within the mouth is more common than externally visible blood.[27] Even in the absence of blood, oral ulcers and bruises are likely painful and are reason to recommend avoiding the use of a bit until the lesion has healed.

Alloys of various metals are used in bits. Oxidation of copper is thought to induce salivation. Titanium is lighter than steel and highly resistant to mechanical damage from the teeth[30] and, although it can cause contact allergy in people, this has not been reported in horses. Nickel causes allergic contact dermatitis in people but the nickel release rate from bits is so small that allergic reactions seem unlikely. However, vesicles on the equine oral mucosae have been reported in response to nickel contact.[30] A current trend is the use of sweet iron bits that develop a blue color after heating to around 300°C. Contact with air and humidity rust the surface giving it a sweet taste that may encourage salivation. The iron released by these bits is below the toxicity level for horses.[30]

CLINICS CARE POINTS

- Saddle fit is not easy to evaluate in the standing horse: it is difficult to assess areas that are hidden from view and back shape changes continuously during locomotion.

- Pay attention to indicators of discomfort that may be related to poorly fitting tack including the horse's facial expression, restricted limb movements and conflict behaviors.

- Adaptations in back shape occur over time in response to the amount and type of exercise; saddle fit needs to be checked regularly and adjusted as necessary to allow the horse to function optimally.

- Innovative equipment does not always function as expected, evaluate on an individual basis.

- If you suspect a horse is suffering from pain related to the bit or bridle, evaluate fit with the tack adjusted in the customary manner. A qualified bit and bridle fitter can be consulted if you are not confident in this area.

DISCLOSURE

Neither of the authors declares any commercial or financial conflicts of interest.

REFERENCES

1. Guire R, Weller R, Fisher M, et al. Investigation Looking at the Repeatability of 20 Society of Master Saddlers Qualified Saddle Fitters' Observations During Static Saddle Fit. J Equine Vet Sci 2017;56:1–5.

2. Murray R, Guire R, Fisher M, et al. Reducing Peak Pressures Under the Saddle Panel at the Level of the 10th to 13th Thoracic Vertebrae May Be Associated With Improved Gait Features, Even When Saddles Are Fitted to Published Guidelines. J Equine Vet Sci 2017;54:60–9.

3. Murray RC, Mackechnie-Guire R, Fisher M, et al. Reducing Peak Pressures Under the Saddle at Thoracic Vertebrae 10-13 is Associated with Alteration in Jump Kinematics. Comp Exerc Physiol 2018;14(4):239–47.

4. Murray R, MacKechnie-Guire R, Fisher M, et al. Could Pressure Distribution Under Race-Exercise Saddles Affect Limb Kinematics and Lumbosacral Flexion in the Galloping Racehorse? J Equine Vet Sci 2019;81:102795.

5. Meschan EM, Peham C, Schobesberger H, et al. The influence of the width of the Saddle Tree on the Forces and the Pressure Distribution Under the Saddle. Vet J 2007;173(3):578–84.

6. Peinen K von, Wiestner T, Rechenberg B von, et al. Relationship Between Saddle Pressure Measurements and Clinical Signs of Saddle Soreness at the withers. Equine Vet J Suppl 2010;(38):650–3.

7. MacKechnie-Guire R, MacKechnie-Guire E, Fairfax V, et al. The Effect of Tree Width on Thoracolumbar and Limb Kinematics, Saddle Pressure Distribution, and Thoracolumbar Dimensions in Sports Horses in Trot and Canter. Animals (Basel) 2019;9(10). https://doi.org/10.3390/ani9100842.

8. Greve L, Dyson SJ. An Investigation of the Relationship between Hindlimb Lameness and Saddle Slip. Equine Vet J 2013;45(5):570–7.

9. Greve L, Dyson SJ. The Interrelationship of Lameness, Saddle Slip and back Shape in the General Sports Horse Population. Equine Vet J 2014;46(6):687–94.

10. Gunst S, Dittmann MT, Arpagaus S, et al. Influence of Functional Rider and Horse Asymmetries on Saddle Force Distribution During Stance and in Sitting Trot. J Equine Vet Sci 2019;78:20–8.

11. Belock B, Kaiser LJ, Lavagnino M, et al. Comparison of Pressure Distribution Under a Conventional Saddle and a Treeless Saddle at Sitting trot. Vet J 2012;193(1):87–91.

12. Hall C, Huws N, White C, et al. Assessment of Ridden Horse Behavior. J Vet Behav 2013;8(2):62–73.

13. Murray R, Guire R, Fisher M, et al. A Bridle Designed to Avoid Peak Pressure Locations Under the Headpiece and Noseband Is Associated With More Uniform Pressure and Increased Carpal and Tarsal Flexion, Compared With the Horse's Usual Bridle. J Equine Vet Sci 2015;35(11–12):947–55.

14. Cross GH, Cheung MK, Honey TJ, et al. Application of a Dual Force Sensor System to Characterize the Intrinsic Operation of Horse Bridles and Bits. J Equine Vet Sci 2017;48:129–35.e3.

15. Uldahl M, Clayton HM. Lesions Associated with the Use of bits, Nosebands, Spurs and Whips in Danish Competition Horses. Equine Vet J 2019;51(2):154–62.

16. Casey V, McGreevy PD, O'Muiris E, et al. A Preliminary Report on Estimating the Pressures Exerted by a Crank Noseband in the Horse. J Vet Behav 2013;8(6):479–84.

17. Doherty O, Conway T, Conway R, et al. An Objective Measure of Noseband Tightness and Its Measurement Using a Novel Digital Tightness Gauge. PLoS One 2017;12(1):e0168996.
18. Clayton HM, Lee R. A Fluoroscopic Study of the position and Action of the jointed Snaffle bit in the Horse's Mouth. J Equine Vet Sci 1984;4(5):193–6.
19. Clayton HM. A Fluoroscopic study of the Position and Action of different bits in the Horse's Mouth. J Equine Vet Sci 1985;5(2):68–77.
20. Manfredi J, Clayton HM, Rosenstein D. Radiographic Study of bit Position within the Horse's Oral Cavity. Equine Comp Exerc Physiol 2005;2(3):195–201.
21. Manfredi JM, Rosenstein D, Lanovaz JL, et al. Fluoroscopic study of oral behaviours in response to the presence of a bit and the effects of rein tension. Comp Exerc Physiol 2009;6(04):143–8.
22. Benoist CC, Cross GH. A Photographic Methodology for Analyzing Bit Position Under Rein Tension. J Equine Vet Sci 2018;67:102–11.
23. Björnsdóttir S, Frey R, Kristjansson T, et al. Bit-related Lesions in Icelandic Competition Horses. Acta Vet Scand 2014;56:40.
24. Uldahl M, Bundegaard L, Dahl J, et al. Assessment of Skin and Mucosa at the Equine Oral Commissures to Assess Pathology from bit wear: The Oral Commissure Assessment Protocol (OCA) for Analysis and Categorisation of Oral Commissures. Animals (Basel) 2022;12(5):643.
25. Uldahl M, Bundgaard L, Dahl J, et al. Pre-Competition Oral Findings in Danish Sport Horses and Ponies Competing at High Level. Animals 2022, 12, 616. https://doi.org/ 10.3390/ani12050616.
26. Tuomola K, Mäki-Kihniä N, Valros A, et al. Bit-Related Lesions in Event Horses After a Cross-Country Test. Front Vet Sci 2021;8:651160.
27. Tuomola K, Mäki-Kihniä N, Kujala-Wirth M, et al. Oral Lesions in the Bit Area in Finnish Trotters After a Race: Lesion Evaluation, Scoring, and Occurrence. Front Vet Sci 2019;6:206.
28. Mata F, Johnson C, Bishop C. A Cross-Sectional Epidemiological Study of Prevalence and Severity of bit-induced Oral Trauma in Polo Ponies and Race Horses. J Appl Anim Welf Sci 2015;18(3):259–68.
29. Engelke E, Gasse H. An Anatomical Study of the Rostral part of the Equine Oral Cavity with Respect to Position and Size of a Snaffle Bit. Equine Vet Educ 2003; 15(3):158–63.
30. Herholz C, Flisch M, Rinaldi D, et al. Metal Analysis of Horse Bits Using X-ray fluoRescence (XRF). PHK 2019;35(3):234–9.
31. Anttila M, Raekallio M, Valros A. Oral Dimensions Related to Bit Size in Adult Horses and Ponies. Front Vet Sci 2022;9:879048.

Managing the Rider

Lesley Goff, PhD, MAnimSt(AnimPhysio), MAppSc(ExSpSc), GDipAppSc(ManipPhysio), BAppSc(Physio)[a,b,*]

KEYWORDS

- Equestrian • Symmetry • Performance • Injury

KEY POINTS

- The rider plays a significant role in equine performance.
- Tactile communication of the rider with the horse can be altered by rider injury or dysfunction.
- Equine practitioners need to consider the rider in cases of poor performance.

 Video content accompanies this article at http://www.vetequine.theclinics. com.

INTRODUCTION

The equestrian sport is unique in that it requires two athletes to work closely together—the horse and the rider. The team must be in absolute harmony to execute even the simplest of maneuvers.[1] There is a large body of evidence that describes the contribution of the rider to not only the movement of the horse but also the performance of the horse, particularly in the thoracolumbar region.[2–4] Unfortunately, specific evaluation of the rider has not been fully incorporated into most diagnostic approaches for assessing poor performance in horses. Veterinarians are limited in their training and scope of practice to evaluating and treating horses and not humans. Therefore, rider assessment needs to become an important part of the overall assessment when managing the horse for any poor performance issue and not just for back pain. Examination of the rider–horse interaction in ridden exercise is multifactorial and includes balance, symmetry, and esthetics of movement. The aim of this article is to give an overview of how the different areas of the rider can affect the horse, using knowledge of biomechanics and evidence where possible. The included images and videos can provide a method to perform a quick screening of the rider to determine if any issues need further evaluation by a registered human professional. Other factors associated with the rider that may affect horse

---

[a] School of Veterinary Science, University of Queensland, Australia; [b] Active Animal Physiotherapy and Hip Sport Spine Physiotherapy, PO Box 277, Highfields, Queensland 4352, Australia
* Corresponding author.
E-mail address: lesley@animalphysio.com.au

Vet Clin Equine 38 (2022) 603–616
https://doi.org/10.1016/j.cveq.2022.07.004
0749-0739/22/© 2022 Elsevier Inc. All rights reserved.

performance include personality traits and the rider's ability to communicate with their horse.[5]

POINTS OF CONTACT

The contact areas of the rider with the horse include (**Figs. 1** and **2**):

- Bony landmarks of the pelvis (seat bones)
- Gluteal musculature
- Pelvic floor musculature
- Medial surfaces of thigh and lower limbs
- Feet
- Hands via the bit

Many other additional areas of the rider's body will also affect the areas directly contacting the horse. These include the ankle, knee, and hip joints; the lumbosacral, thoracic, and cervical regions; and the shoulder, elbow, and wrists.

In ridden equine sports, the rider provides signals to communicate with the horse, which can be considered a tactile interchange of information between the rider and the horse.[6] The contact areas of the rider that provide direct communication with the horse are regions of the pelvis and legs, and indirectly by the hands via bit contact. It would make sense that symmetrical contact of these areas of the rider with the horse would be ideal. However this may not always be the case. The skill of the rider can obviously affect horse performance, but here we will be addressing rider symmetry, which can be influenced by physical injuries and impairments of the rider.

ASSESSING THE RIDER

When assessing how a horse performs, particularly if the reason for poor performance is difficult to diagnose, it is often useful to observe the horse being ridden. Some conditions in the horse, such as thoracolumbar and sacroiliac joint pain, seem to be made worse by the presence of a rider.[7] This could be a factor of the rider's weight, as there

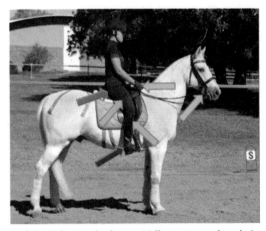

Fig. 1. Contact areas of the rider on the horse. Yellow arrows: hand via the bit. Crimson arrow: gluteal musculature. Green arrows: musculature of the inner thigh and medial lower limb. Purple arrow: ankle/foot. Other areas are shown diagrammatically in **Fig. 2**.

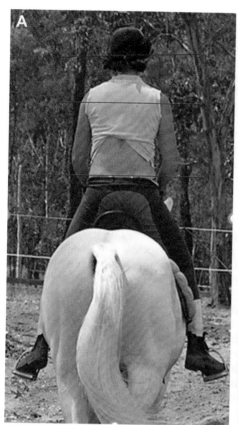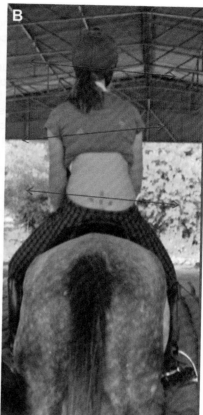

Fig. 2. Illustration of contact areas of the pelvis with the horse that are unable to be viewed in vivo. Pubic symphysis (*A*) and ramus (*B*) are shown in the lateral view in the left drawing. Ischial tuberosities (seat bones) are shown from the caudal view in the right drawing.

has been an association with heavier riders and induced lameness.[8] However, riders themselves have injuries, asymmetries, and impairments which can affect how they physically communicate with the horse. Even in the absence of injuries, rider asymmetries in the hip and pelvic area[9] and leg length may have an impact on equestrian performance. Regardless of rider skill or horse ability, pre-existing rider injuries or dysfunction, which may include scoliosis, back or pelvic pain, neck or shoulder pain, hip, knee, or ankle stiffness, and leg length difference, may exist. The role of the equine practitioner is to take the history of the current complaint regarding the horse and ask about the presence of current or past conditions in the rider. Some of these conditions are magnified with rider aging, especially arthropathies, and affect the ability of the rider to maintain balanced contact and move in synchrony with the horse. Musculoskeletal injuries and asymmetries may also affect the ability of the rider's neuromotor control, which may hamper the ability to produce the skilled movements required for communication with the horse.

When clinical signs in the horse are exacerbated by riding exercise as opposed to in-hand or lunging, saddle fit, rider skill, and rider weight must be considered. The rider may be tactfully advised regarding such issues. The rider may be tactfully advised regarding such issues. It may also be useful to observe the rider on the ground to observe any obvious postural asymmetries. This can be done by looking at the rider standing on level ground or if a leg length difference is suspected, then observed, and measured while lying on a flat surface or while sitting on a saddle barrel or saddle chair (**Fig. 3**).

In riders with less visually obvious issues, it is useful to place sticky dots on relevant body landmarks to make visualization of postural or movement asymmetries easier (**Fig. 4**A, B). This should be done on a level surface where possible. It is frequently beneficial for the rider to see themselves in either still images or video footage to understand how their impairment and postural issues may be negatively affecting the horse. The rider can then be encouraged to have these issues addressed by an appropriately qualified practitioner. This can assist the practitioner to decide if there are static or dynamic components of the rider that are adversely affecting horse performance.

A drop of the rider's pelvis to one side and a tilting of the rider's upper body to one side (**Fig. 5**A, B) are considered physical factors that contribute to asymmetrical saddle pressures.[2] How these issues are addressed is complex as they often involve concurrent asymmetries in the horse[2] and saddle displacement during mounting from one side.[10] The practitioner needs to use clinical reasoning and a methodical approach to assess each potential factor that might be contributing to poor performance issues.

One of the most commonly reported rider injuries is low back pain.[11] However, there is often no conclusive MRI evidence to suggest that the source of the back pain is because of overt lumbar spine pathology.[12] Most kinematic studies of riders focus on trunk, pelvic, and lumbosacral movements, but other regions of the body are also important to assess for total integration of the rider with the horse. It cannot be stressed enough that even though certain regions of the rider's body may appear to be more clinically relevant, it is important to look at the rider as a whole entity.

PELVIS AND LUMBAR SPINE

The position and movement of the rider's pelvis are important to consider as they provide a key role in communication with the horse. Peham and colleagues (2010)[3] describe the stable seat as a foundation on which effective communication is based,

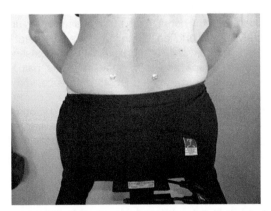

Fig. 3. Rider sitting on a saddle chair on a level surface. Dots have been placed on two of the pelvic bony landmarks to assist with visualizing the slight pelvic tilt (higher on the right side) and slight left lateral curve of the lumbar spine.

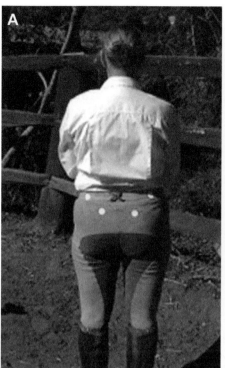 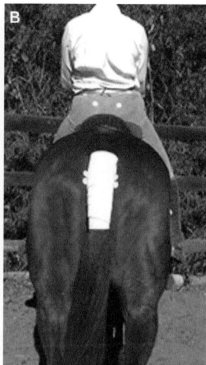

Fig. 4. (A, B) Observation of the rider while standing and mounted. The rider (A) has dots placed on the posterior aspect of the iliac crest and the posterior superior iliac spines of the pelvis, which appear to be relatively level. In contrast, when mounted (B) the dots reveal a relative tilting and rotation of the pelvis to the left. It is not readily apparent if these changes are because of the saddle, the rider, or the horse, or a combination of all three without further assessment of all the associated factors.

with riders being required to adapt temporally and spatially to the movement of the horse's trunk to keep a well-adjusted seat. Adapting to the horse's movements requires a gait-specific motion of the rider's pelvis.[13]

The contact points of the pelvis with the saddle induce local forces that are transferred upward and absorbed in other parts of the rider's body (see **Fig. 2**). The rider's sacroiliac joint transfers these forces from the bones of the pelvis via the lumbosacral joint, to the lumbar spine and trunk. Even though it is important for load transfer, the range of joint motion at the rider's sacroiliac joint is small. Much of the adaptation of the rider to the horse's movements occurs at the lumbosacral junction and the hip joints. The lumbosacral and hip articulations have larger ranges of joint motion compared with the sacroiliac joint, and therefore can be readily visualized and assessed for motion during assessment of the rider (**Fig. 6**, Video 1).

There is generally more sagittal movement of the pelvis than at the trunk,[14] and posterior pelvic rotation coupled with flexion of the lumbar spine is required for the rider to perform collection and movements such as piaffe and passage in dressage.[15] The lumbosacral joint must move well to accommodate pelvic motion, and thus it is important to observe, regarding movement and control. A rider with arthropathy, pain or limitation of motion at the lumbosacral junction and, to an extent, the more cranial lumbar

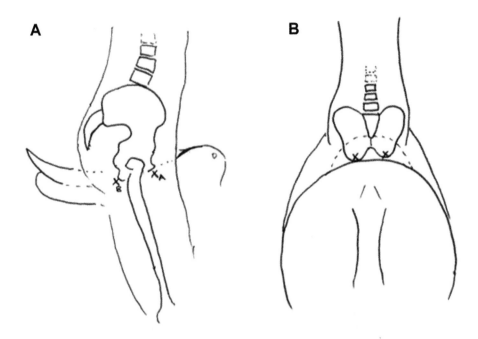

Fig. 5. (*A, B*) Observation of differences in rider's posture while riding. Despite being photo-graphed in rising trot, the rider on the left (*A*) is a more balanced (indicated by horizontal lines drawn at the levels of the occiput, just below spine of scapulae and the level of the posterior superior iliac spines of the pelvis). The rider on the right (*B*) has lines drawn to indi-cate the levels of the occiput, the inferior scapular angles, and posterior superior iliac spines of the pelvis. There is the appearance of pelvis tilted down to the right, a difference in po-sition of the scapulae with right scapula appearing more cranial, and protracted (forward positioned) hence why the line does not appear to correspond to the yellow dot on that side. This forward position of right shoulder girdle combines with left trunk rotation. This altered posture also causes the knee and heel height appear to be unleveled, and the rider appears to have her head rotated toward the right, possibly to center her eyes and compen-sate for the relative left rotation of the trunk.

articulations, will be affected in how they position the pelvis in a sagittal plane and into rotation and lateral tilt. The ability to position the pelvis via the lumbosacral junction can be assessed with the rider sitting on the horse, or on a saddle stand with saddle (Video 2). If the rider cannot achieve pelvic positioning (anterior and posterior rotation, or tilt) via manual guidance or verbal cues, then liaising with a human musculoskeletal practitioner is required.

It is also useful to consider that forces from the pelvic contact points (see **Fig. 2**) are symmetrically transmitted through the rider's pelvis. Although not directly in contact with the saddle, the rider's iliac crests are readily palpated and, if asymmetrical, could indicate acquired or inherent pelvic asymmetry in the rider (**Fig. 7**A).

The muscles of the pelvic floor form an important component of the core stability muscles in riders. These muscles are often in direct contact with the saddle. There may be a relationship between good pelvic floor function and riding.[16] It may be impor-tant for riders, especially post-partum and peri-menopausal women, or male riders who have had surgery or intervention for prostate dysfunction, to have their pelvic floor function assessed by a pelvic floor practitioner.

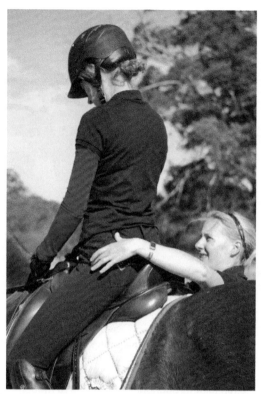

Fig. 6. Assessing the rider's lumbosacral movement and motor control using verbal and manual cues for anterior and posterior pelvic tilt (relative extension and flexion at the lumbosacral junction). The assessor asks the rider to rotate or tilt the pelvis anteriorly and then posteriorly, with gentle manual guidance from the therapist's hands to assist the movement.

HIP JOINT

Hip movement may be considered as movement of the femur relative to the fixed acetabulum of the pelvis or movement of the pelvis over the fixed femoral head. Both aspects of this movement are important for the subtle positioning of the rider's pelvis. Delivery of subtle leg movements for communication by the rider is dictated by both hip mobility and muscle function at the hip joint. The muscles involved in hip movement and positioning of the whole lower limb are the adductors (adductors longus, magnus, brevis, pectineus, gracilis) and abductors of the thigh (gluteus medius, gluteus minimus, and tensor fascia lata), hip extensors (gluteus maximus, hamstrings, posterior head of adductor magnus), and flexors (rectus femoris, psoas major and iliacus). Some of these muscles also rotate the hip (glutei, psoas major), as do the piriformis and sartorius. The muscles involved in stability of the hip tend to be smaller and closer to the joint and include the quadratus femoris, gluteus minimus, gemelli, and obturators—often referred to as deep hip stabilizers. These muscles have a role in stabilizing the hip and pelvis. Hip extension and external rotation are considered important components in riding.[9,17] Hip movements of the rider can be assessed on the horse with the feet in or out of the stirrups (**Fig. 8**) but are more easily assessed off-horse. Observation of the ability of the rider to actively move and for the practitioner

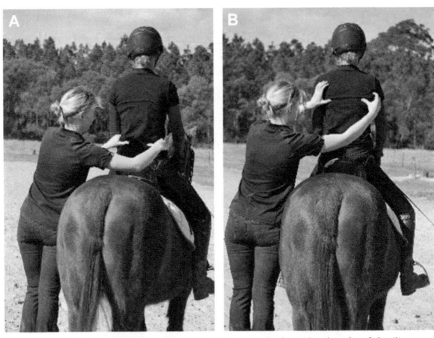

Fig. 7. (*A, B*) Assessing the rider's posture via palpating the bony landmarks of the iliac crests of the pelvis (*A*) and the inferior angles of the scapulae (*B*).

to passively move the hip joint throughout its full range of motion is useful for assessing muscle and joint function (see Video 2; Videos 3 and 4). Hip movements are also suggested as a useful screening test for riders who may suffer from low back pain.[18]

Conditions which may limit hip joint mobility include osteoarthritis, labral tears, femoroacetabular impingement, gluteal tendinopathy, and conditions secondary to lumbopelvic disorders.[19] Primary conditions of the hip often result in an adductor–abductor muscle imbalance where the abductors tend to become underactive and the adductors tend to be more readily recruited.[20] Hip joint pain and pathology can induce inhibition of the muscles that stabilize the hip.[21] Proper assessment of hip

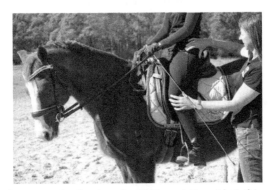

Fig. 8. Assessing the amount of external rotation at the rider's hip when the rider is mounted. The clinician's right hand is assessing movement near the hip at the top of the thigh with the left hand guiding active seated external rotation at the level of the knee.

function by a qualified musculoskeletal practitioner is imperative for optimal communication between the rider's legs and the horse.

TRUNK AND SHOULDER

The rider's trunk position will dictate the position of their neck and shoulders. Positional or postural rotations of the trunk affect positioning of the rider's shoulder via the scapulothoracic articulation. Assessment of the position of the rider's scapulae can be readily accomplished via direct palpation (**Fig. 7**B). Assessing the ability of the rider to rotate their trunk to the right and left, both on and off the horse, can highlight a cause for the appearance of shoulder height differences or forward-backward (protraction-retraction) positioning of the shoulder. This appearance is often due to the rider's positioning of the scapulothoracic articulation to accommodate for the limitation of trunk rotation or thoracolumbar region stiffness (**Fig. 9**). Assessing the ability of the rider to laterally bend the trunk to the left and right can highlight vertebral segment limitations and myofascial limitations to movement (Video 5).

Trunk position can be affected by structural and functional injuries or impairments in the thoracolumbar region, which include scoliosis, spondylosis, and motor control deficits in the adjacent spinal musculature. The iliopsoas, abdominals, respiratory muscles, latissimus dorsi, serratus anterior, erector spinae, thoracolumbar fascia, pectorals, rhomboids, and trapezius and can affect the ability of the trunk to rotate, laterally bend, and extend. Trunk mobility and positioning may also be affected by rider handedness as some of these muscles are used for habitual positioning of the hand and upper limb for daily tasks. Activation of the rider's trunk musculature is important to help ameliorate the perturbations transferred to the rider by the horse, and to maintain posture and minimize movement of the rider's arms and legs.[22] Trunk position and range of motion may be improved by local articular mobilization or manipulation and stretching of the musculature.

Scoliosis of the thoracolumbar region can be because of either structural or functional defects. In structural scoliosis, vertebral defects that induce abnormal rotation and lateral curvatures do not self-correct or straighten out when the rider bends over to their toes (Video 6). Functional scoliosis is due to left-right muscle imbalances, and the observed rotation and lateral curvature are abolished when the rider bends forward to touch their toes. Functional scoliosis may be altered by targeted stretching.

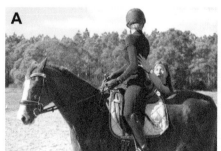 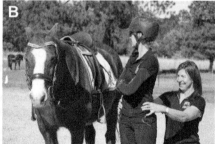

Fig. 9. (*A, B*) Assessing rider's trunk rotation off (*A*) and on the horse (*B*). In (*A*) the rider is standing with feet hip width apart and the clinician stabilizes the pelvis lightly and asks the rider to rotate trunk toward the right. Pattern of movement is noted by the clinician and then compared with rotation to the left. In (*B*) the rider is asked to rotate toward the right, keeping pelvis still in the saddle. Here the clinician is guiding the rider gently into trunk rotation. Pattern of rotation is felt/observed and then compared with rotation to the left.

Surface EMG analysis can be used to assess the ability of the rider to adjust the position of their trunk and, through this, affect the movement of the horse. Experienced riders use their rectus abdominis muscles to induce trunk flexion. In contrast to novice riders, who coactivate their rectus abdominis and iliocostalis lumborum muscles—a less energy efficient activation strategy—experienced riders activate their rectus abdominus muscles more efficiently and controlledly. Age may be an additional factor affecting the control strategy of the trunk muscles, with older riders less able to activate selectively their rectus abdominus without iliocostalis lumborum contraction to produce trunk flexion. Further research is needed to investigate the relationship between the rider's control of muscle activity and how it is reflected in the horse's performance.[23]

KNEE AND ANKLE

The movements of the ankle, knee, hip, and lumbosacral articulations are coupled in the rider. Disciplines, such as show-jumping and flat racing that are ridden using a short stirrup position require more flexion at the rider's hip, knee, and ankle, compared with dressage or other forms of riding that require a straighter lower limb. Maintaining adequate knee and ankle joint range of motion in riders involved in show jumping is critical to allowing the rider greater impulsion in the initial phase of the jump and provides better shock absorption for the rider when landing.[18] Some research suggests that there is no effect of rider position on horse jumping kinematics or motion,[24] so adequate lower limb angles for riders involved in those shorter-stirrup disciplines may only be important for positioning the rider's body as required for jumping or flat racing.

A recent study has suggested that reduced joint range of motion during knee flexion and hip adduction in riders may be a predictor of the development of low back pain.[18] In the same study, the authors report that there is a good correlation between hip and knee joint range of motion and the effect the movement at those two joints has on the sagittal position of the lumbopelvic region in the rider. The amount of knee flexion and extension that occurs during riding is reduced in skilled riders, which improves the rider's ability to synchronize with the motion of the horse.[15] This suggests that it is important for riders to develop good motor control of lower limb muscles to limit extraneous limb motion.

The ability of the rider to achieve ankle dorsiflexion (angles less than 90 degrees) with the foot positioned in a stirrup is a requirement in most riding disciplines. Ankle mobility in dorsiflexion may be limited by joint stiffness (e.g., osteoarthritis) or shortening of the muscles responsible for ankle flexion. Assessing dorsiflexion of the rider's ankle may be done when mounted in a stirrup or off the horse (**Fig. 10**).

ELBOW AND WRIST

The ability to maintain consistent contact with the bit during all phases of the different gaits is necessary to facilitate good rider–horse communication. Elbow and shoulder joint movements are important in riding to enable consistency of contact. Terada (2006)[25] reported that coordinated flexion-extension of the shoulder and elbow joints was required in skilled riders, so that a constant distance from the rider's wrist to the bit was maintained despite variation in range of motion of the shoulders or hip articulations. Controlled arm movements are coordinated by activation of the rider's biceps brachii and triceps brachii to control motion at the elbow joint.[25]

HEAD AND NECK

Significant trunk rotation causes changes in the head and neck positions in an effort to maintain the rider's vision directed forward in the direction of travel (see **Fig. 3**). In a

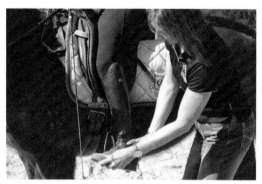

Fig. 10. Assessing the range of dorsiflexion at the rider's ankle. The clinician is guiding the rider into dorsiflexion. Angles of 90 degrees and less are desirable for all riding disciplines.

kinematic study of elite riders, head movements were very small compared with the movements of other body segments.[14] This suggests that muscular control of the head and neck is important. Riders with neck pain or stiffness may have reduced muscle control of the head or neck and may not be able to stabilize or coordinate head and neck movements.[26] Affected riders may compensate by changing their shoulder or trunk position and may be unable to position their eyes level and their heads facing forward for optimal performance. Riders with a history of neck pain and stiffness should be assessed by an appropriately qualified practitioner.

GENERAL PRACTICAL GUIDELINES FOR RIDERS

A program that focuses on flexibility is recommended as part of a physical fitness plan for riders.[18] Riders may participate in specific flexibility programs designed by exercise physiologists, physiotherapists, or riding coaches based on the results of screening or where there are known injuries and impairments. Riders may also participate in a more generalized flexibility program, such as yoga. There are several online resources for yoga practices designed for riders. However, most scientific literature reports on exercises designed to improve flexibility focus on measures of pain and quality of life and not specifically on improvements in joint mobility or flexibility.[27–29]

Muscle activation and coordination of the rider is required to adequately position the pelvis, trunk, and limbs during different gaits or athletic activities to minimize the mechanical forces transferred from the horse to the rider.[17] Motor patterns that are disrupted by pain and dysfunction may be addressed by qualified practitioners, such as physiotherapists and exercise physiologists, or more generally by pilates, which should be directed by a properly qualified pilates instructor. There is evidence to suggest that equipment-based pilates exercise is better than pilates based on matwork for the management of low back pain.[30] Most of the reviews on the efficacy of pilates are promising for addressing low back pain but do not address athletic performance.[31]

SUMMARY

There is an undeniable effect of the rider on horse performance as the rider forms an integral component of the horse–rider interaction. Few equine practitioners may have a background in human medicine and health care, and therefore, most veterinarians have a limited understanding of how to formally assess rider impairments and asymmetries. Equine practitioners with a riding background often have more personal knowledge of the biomechanics of riding and the importance of horse–rider interactions. It is good practice to ask riders if they have any significant musculoskeletal or neurologic injuries, either current or past, that they feel may negatively affect their horse's performance. If the rider has already sought out professional advice or treatment, it is important for the equine practitioner to collaborate, when possible, to discuss issues related to the horse–rider interaction.

CLINICS CARE POINTS

- Equine performance may be affected by the rider, so rider exercise is needed to fully assess horse–rider interactions.
- Riders need to be asked about their injuries as they relate to their horse's performance.
- Practitioners can do a quick screening of the rider on the ground and on the horse by using a few simple techniques.
- Riders with injuries or obvious asymmetry or dysfunction should be directed to an appropriately qualified human practitioner for diagnosis and ongoing management.
- Open communication with the human practitioner about a rider's injuries or impairments is a useful part of the management of performance problems in horses.
- When assessing the rider, it is always best to ask for permission to physically touch or examine the rider.

DISCLOSURE

The author has nothing to disclose.

SUPPLEMENTARY DATA

Supplementary data related to this article can be found online at https://doi.org/10.1016/j.cveq.2022.07.004.

REFERENCES

1. Sorli J. Equestrian injuries: a five year review of hospital admissions in British Columbia, Canada. Inj Prev 2000;6:59–61.
2. Gunst S, Dittman M, Arpagaus S, et al. Influence of functional rider and horse asymmetries on saddle force distribution in stance and during sitting trot. JEVS 2019;78:20–8.
3. Peham C, Kotschwar A, Borkenhagen B, et al. A comparison of forces acting on the horse's back and the stability of the rider's seat in different positions at the trot. Vet J 2010;184:56–9.
4. MacKechnie-Guire R, MacKechnie-Guire E, Fairfax V, et al. The effect that induced rider asymmetry has on equine locomotion and the range of motion of the thoracolumbar spine when ridden in rising trot. JEVS 2020;88:102946.
5. McGowan C, Hyytiainen H. Muscular and neuromotor control and learning in the athletic horse. Comp Ex Phys 2017;13:185–94.
6. Munz A, Eckhadt F, Witte K. Horse-rider interaction in dressage riding. Hum Mov Sci 2014;33:226–37.
7. Barstow A, Dyson S. Clinical features and diagnosis of sacroiliac joint region pain in 296 horses: 2004-2014. Equine Vet Educ 2015;27:637–47.

8. Dyson S, Ellis A, MacKechnie-Guire R, et al. The influence of rider:horse body-weight ratio and rider-horse-saddle fit on equine gait and behaviour: A pilot study. Eq Vet Educ 2020;32:527–39.

9. Gandy E, Bondi A, Hogg R, et al. A preliminary investigation in the use of inertial sensing technology for the measurement of hip rotation asymmetry in horse riders. Sports Technol 2014;7:79–88.

10. Geutjens C, Clayton H, Kaiser I. Forces and pressure beneath the saddle during mounting from the ground and from a raised mounting platform. Vet J 2008;175:332–7.

11. Quinn S, Bird S. Influence of saddle type on the incidence of lower back pain in equestrian riders. Br J Sports Med 1986;30:140–4.

12. Kraft C, Pennekamp P, Becker U, et al. Magnetic resonance imaging findings of the lumbar spine in elite horseback riders. Am J Sports Med 2009;37:2205–13.

13. Symes D, Ellis E. A preliminary study of rider asymmetry within equitation. Vet J 2009;181:34–7.

14. Eckhardt F, Munz A, Witte K. Application of a full body inertial system in dressage riding. JEVS 2014;34:1294–9.

15. Bystrom A, Roepstroff L, Geser-von-Peinen K, et al. Differences in rider movement pattern between different degrees of collection at the trot in high-level dressage horses ridden on a treadmill. Hum Mov Sci 2015;41:1–8.

16. Carboni C, Blanquet M, Jaramillo K. Effectiveness of Horseback Riding in the Management of Pelvic Floor Dysfunctions. Int J Health Rehab Sci 2014. https://doi.org/10.5455/ijhrs.000000045.

17. Baxter J, Hobbs S, Alexander J. Rider skill affects time and frequency domain postural variables when performing shoulder-in. J Equine Vet Sci 2022. https://doi.org/10.1016/j.jevs.2021.103805.

18. Cejudo A, Gines-Diaz A, de Baranda P. Asymmetry and tightness of lower limb muscles in equestrian athletes: are they predictors for back pain? Symmetry 2020;12:1679.

19. Reiman M, Matheson L. Restricted hip mobility: Clinical suggestions for self-mobilization and muscle re-education. Int J Sp Phys Ther 2013;8:729–40.

20. Allison K, Vicenzino B, Wrigley T, et al. Hip abductor muscle weakness in individuals with gluteal tendinopathy. Med Sci Sports Exerc 2016;48:346–52.

21. Retchford T, Crossley K, Grimaldi A, et al. Can local muscles augment stability in the hip? A narrative literature review. J Musculoskelet Neuronal Interact 2013;13:1–12.

22. Terada K, Mullineaux D, Lanovaz J, et al. Electromyographic analysis of the rider's muscles at trot. Equine Comp Exerc Physiol 2007;1:193–8.

23. Pantall A, Barton S, Collins P. Surface electromyography of abdominal and spinal muscles in adult horse riders during rising trot. In: Harrison A, Anderson R, Kenny I, editors. ISBS 27 International symposium on biomechanics in sports. Limerick; 2009.

24. Power P, Harrison A. Influences of a rider on the rotation of the horse-rider system during jumping. Equine Comp Exerc Physiol 2004;1:33–40.

25. Terada K, Clayton H, Kato K. Stabilization of wrist position during horseback riding at trot. Equine Comp Exerc Physiol 2006;3:179–84.

26. Treleaven J. Sensorimotor disturbances in neck disorders, affecting postural stability head and eye movement control. Man Ther 2008;13:2–11.

27. Cramer H, Lauche R, Haller H, et al. A systematic review and meta-analysis of yoga for low back pain. Clin J Pain 2013;29:450–60.

28. Geneen L, Moore R, Clarke C, et al. Physical activity and exercise for chronic pain in adults: an overview of Cochrane Reviews. Cochrane Database Syst Rev 2017; 24:CD011279.

29. Owen P, Miller C, Mundell N, et al. Which specific modes of exercise are most effective for treating low back pain? Network meta-analysis. Br J Sports Med 2020;54:1279–87.

30. da Luz M, Pena Costa L, Fuhro F, et al. Effectiveness of mat Pilates or equipment-based Pilates exercises in patients with chronic nonspecific low back pain: a randomized controlled trial. Phys Ther 2014;94:623–31.

31. Miyamoto G, Costa L, Cabral C. Efficacy of the Pilates method for pain and disability in patients with chronic nonspecific low back pain: a systematic review with meta-analysis. Braz J Phys Ther 2013;17:517–32.

Printed and bound by CPI Group (UK) Ltd, Croydon, CR0 4YY

03/10/2024

01040481-0014